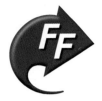

Fast Facts

CW00537572

Fast Facts.
Acute Coronary
Syndromes

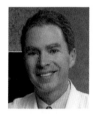

Paul A Gurbel MD FACC FAHA
Director
Sinai Center for Thrombosis Research
Sinai Hospital
Baltimore, USA

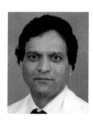

Udaya S Tantry PhD
Laboratory Director
Sinai Center for Thrombosis Research
Sinai Hospital
Baltimore, USA

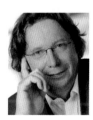

Kurt Huber MD FESC FACC
Director
3rd Department of Medicine
Cardiology and Emergency Medicine
Wilhelminenhospital
Vienna, Austria

Declaration of Independence
This book is as balanced and as practical as we can make it.
Ideas for improvement are always welcome: feedback@fastfacts.com

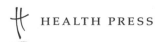

HEALTH PRESS

Fast Facts: Acute Coronary Syndromes
First edition January 2014

Text © 2014 Paul A Gurbel, Udaya S Tantry, Kurt Huber
© 2014 in this edition Health Press Limited

Health Press Limited, Elizabeth House, Queen Street, Abingdon,
Oxford OX14 3LN, UK
Tel: +44 (0)1235 523233
Fax: +44 (0)1235 523238

Book orders can be placed by telephone or via the website.
For regional distributors or to order via the website, please go to: fastfacts.com
For telephone orders, please call +44 (0)1752 202301 (UK, Europe and
Asia–Pacific), 1 800 247 6553 (USA, toll free) or +1 419 281 1802 (Americas).

Fast Facts is a trademark of Health Press Limited.

A CIP record for this title is available from the British Library.

ISBN 978-1-908541-47-5

Gurbel PA (Paul)
Fast Facts: Acute Coronary Syndromes/
Paul A Gurbel, Udaya S Tantry, Kurt Huber

Cover: colored angiogram showing a severe blockage in the
left anterior descending artery of a patient with an acute
coronary syndrome.

Medical illustrations by Annamaria Dutto, Withernsea, UK.
Typesetting and page layout by Zed, Oxford, UK.
Printed by Latimer Trend & Company, Plymouth, UK.

Text printed on biodegradable and recyclable paper
manufactured using elemental chorine free (ECF) wood
pulp from well-managed forests.

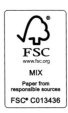

FSC
www.fsc.org

MIX

Paper from
responsible sources
FSC® C013436

List of abbreviations

ACE: angiotensin-converting enzyme

ACS: acute coronary syndromes

ADP: adenosine diphosphate

ARB: angiotensin receptor blocker

ASA: acetylsalicylic acid (aspirin)

BNP: B-type natriuretic peptide

CABG: coronary artery bypass grafting

CAD: coronary artery disease

CAM: cell adhesion molecule

CK-MB: creatine kinase, myocardial band form

COX: cyclo-oxygenase

CRP: C-reactive protein

CT: computed tomography

CYPs: cytochromes

DAPT: dual antiplatelet therapy

DOAC: direct oral anticoagulant

ECG: electrocardiogram

FMC: first medical contact

GP: glycoprotein

GRACE: Global Registry of Acute Coronary Events (risk score)

INR: international normalized ratio

LBBB: left bundle branch block

LDL: low density lipoprotein (cholesterol)

LMWH: low-molecular-weight heparin

LV: left ventricular

MI: myocardial infarction

MMP: matrix metalloproteinase

MRI: magnetic resonance imaging

NSAIDs: non-steroidal anti-inflammatory drugs

NSTEMI: non-ST-segment elevation myocardial infarction

NT-pro-BNP: N-terminal prohormone fragment of BNP

PCI: percutaneous coronary intervention

PPI: proton-pump inhibitor

RBBB: right bundle branch block

ROS: reactive oxygen species

SDNN: standard deviation of normal to normal RR interval

STEMI: ST-segment elevation myocardial infarction

TIMI: Thrombolysis in Myocardial Infarction (risk score)

t-PA: tissue-type plasminogen activator

Tx: thromboxane

UA: unstable angina

UH: unfractionated heparin

URL: upper reference limit (upper limit of normal)

Introduction

Significant changes in socioeconomic status and lifestyle in developing countries, and the rise in prevalence of major risk factors such as obesity, diabetes and advanced age, have led to a significant increase in the prevalence of cardiovascular disease; it is estimated to become the leading cause of death and disability worldwide by the year 2020. Consequently, many countries have instituted counseling and educational methods to encourage people to reduce their risks for developing heart disease. The atherosclerotic process *can* be attenuated effectively and its consequences markedly reduced, with proper preventive measures. Continued efforts in primary and secondary prevention and better understanding and education of cardiovascular risk factors are critical in order to improve cardiac health.

Acute coronary syndromes (ACS) constitute a major part of cardiovascular disease. In recent years, significant improvements have been made in our understanding of the pathophysiology of ACS. Potent pharmacological agents and innovative invasive treatment strategies have been developed, and awareness of secondary treatment strategies has increased. These factors have led to a higher rate of adherence and improved short-term clinical outcomes. Furthermore, improved reperfusion strategies and innovative pharmacological therapies have steadily reduced mortality. Nevertheless, ACS is still a major cause for acute hospitalizations, and the long-term event rate remains high.

Fast Facts: Acute Coronary Syndromes is an international evidence-based primer that will familiarize healthcare professionals with the pathophysiology and clinical presentation of ACS. Importantly, it focuses on the key factors that will optimize patient outcomes, namely accurate initial diagnosis, appropriate risk stratification, and proper therapeutic decision-making in line with both American and European management guidelines. It provides comprehensive and up-to-date information on the available technologies and treatment strategies, along with an overview of novel ideas that are likely to be implemented in the near future, with the ultimate aim of assisting best practice in the identification and management of all patients with ACS.

There are three types of acute coronary syndrome (ACS), defined by the presence or absence of cardiac marker elevation and characteristic ECG changes:
- unstable angina (UA)
- non-ST-segment elevation myocardial infarction (NSTEMI)
- ST-segment elevation myocardial infarction (STEMI).

Myocardial infarction (MI) is a manifestation of ACS and is pathologically defined as myocardial cell death due to prolonged ischemia. All types of ACS are usually associated with chest pain or at least chest discomfort.

Although some pathological findings are shared by each entity, they differ in clinical severity. UA is characterized by an absence of biomarkers in the circulation, whereas MI results in the release of biomarkers into the circulation such as cardiac-specific troponins T or I, or cardiac-specific fraction of creatine kinase (CK)-MB. NSTEMI results from a partial (or a transient but complete) coronary occlusion and distal embolization of platelet-fibrin thrombi, compromising microcirculatory blood flow. These patients have acute chest pain but without persistent ST-segment elevation. STEMI results from a sudden and complete occlusion of an epicardial artery, and these patients have persistent (> 20 minutes) ST-segment elevation, indicative of transmural ischemia. Distal embolization can also occur in STEMI. Figures 1.1 and 1.2 provide an overview of the full spectrum of ACS and the characteristic features of each entity.

Atherosclerotic plaque formation

Pathological and imaging observations indicate that the common underlying mechanism of ACS is atherosclerotic plaque rupture or erosion followed by superimposed thrombosis formation and distal embolization. These processes result in myocardial hypoperfusion. Atherosclerosis is a chronic inflammatory disease involving large and medium-sized arteries. Although it begins early in life, the speed of progression is non-linear, unpredictable and varies markedly between individuals.

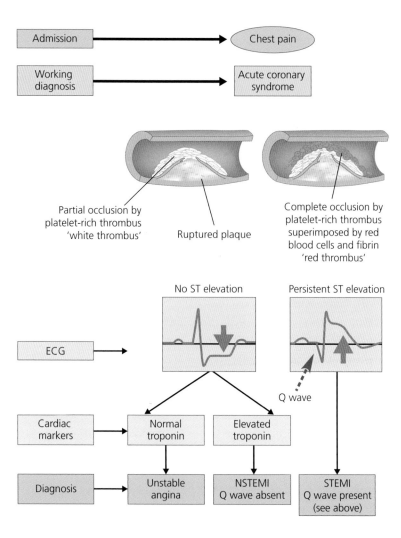

Figure 1.1 The spectrum of acute coronary syndromes, as defined by the degree of coronary occlusion (see also Figure 1.2), characteristic ECG changes (pink arrows indicate presence or absence of ST elevation; dotted blue arrow shows presence of Q wave) and the presence or absence of biomarkers in the circulation. NSTEMI, non-ST-segment elevation myocardial infarction; STEMI, ST-segment elevation myocardial infarction.

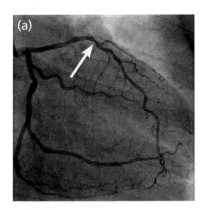

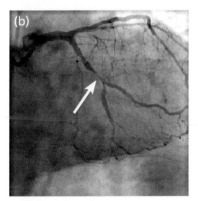

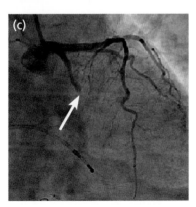

Figure 1.2 Coronary angiography provides detailed structural information that allows an assessment of prognosis and provides direction for appropriate management. Angiograms for (a) unstable angina. The arrow indicates narrowing in the mid left anterior descending artery; (b) non-ST-segment elevation myocardial infarction (NSTEMI). The arrow indicates narrowing of the coronary artery; and (c) ST-segment elevation myocardial infarction (STEMI). The arrow indicates occlusion of the coronary artery.

Dysfunctional endothelium. Atherosclerosis starts with the development of dysfunctional endothelium in the presence of cardiovascular risk factors (Table 1.1).

Under normal conditions, healthy vascular endothelium prevents adhesion of platelets to the endothelium and platelet activation by producing antithrombotic factors, including ectoADPase (CD39), prostaglandin I_2, nitric oxide, matrix metalloproteinase (MMP)-9, protein S, thrombomodulin and tissue-type plasminogen activator (t-PA). However, in the presence of numerous risk factors (see Table 1.1), the normal endothelium loses its antithrombotic properties, which results in the generation of dysfunctional enodothelium.

Dysfunctional endothelium is characterized by vasoconstriction, a proatherogenic environment and increased expression of proinflammatory selectins and cell adhesion molecules (CAMs). These molecules facilitate the binding and internalization of monocytes into the subendothelial space where they transform into macrophages. Moreover, changes in endothelial permeability and the composition of the subendothelial matrix facilitate the entry and retention of cholesterol-rich low-density lipoprotein (LDL) particles.

The macrophages avidly engulf the LDL cholesterol and transform into foam cells, leading to the formation of yellow fatty streaks. This last process further enhances the activation and recruitment

TABLE 1.1

Risk factors for atherosclerosis

Traditional risk factors	Non-traditional risk factors
• Increased age	• Shear stress
• Diabetes mellitus	• Systemic inflammation
• Smoking	• Oxidative stress
• Hypertension	• Advanced glycation end products
• Hyperlipidemia	
• Genetic abnormalities	• Homocysteinemia
• Renal dysfunction	• Immunosuppressive therapy

of inflammatory cells and smooth muscle cells, and the inflamed endothelial cells further promote the adhesion and activation of platelets. Activated platelets serve as inflammatory mediators by expressing various membrane receptors capable of interacting with leukocytes and endothelial cells and thereby significantly contributing to the progression of atherosclerosis (Figures 1.3 and 1.4).

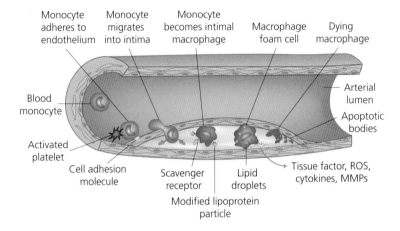

Figure 1.3 Atherosclerosis. Normal endothelium resists prolonged contact with leukocytes, including blood monocytes. However, activated platelets roll along the endothelium, induce a proatherogenic environment and recruit circulating blood monocytes. Cell adhesion molecules associated with the dysfunctional endothelium facilitate the binding and internalization of monocytes into the subendothelial space where they transform into macrophages. The macrophages express scavenger receptors that avidly bind internalized low-density lipoprotein (LDL) particles, and transform into foam cells, a hallmark of the arterial lesion. They are named because of their foamy appearance under the microscope, which is the result of accumulation of lipid droplets within the cytoplasm. The foam cells secrete proinflammatory cytokines that amplify the local inflammatory response in the lesion, as well as reactive oxygen species (ROS). Eventually the macrophages congregate in a central core in the typical atherosclerotic plaque. Macrophages can die in this location, some by apoptosis, hence producing the so-called 'necrotic core' of the atherosclerotic lesion. MMP, matrix metalloproteinase.

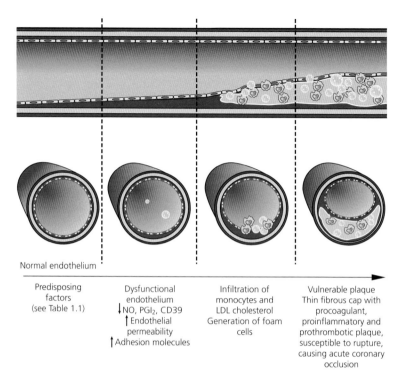

Normal endothelium

| Predisposing factors (see Table 1.1) | Dysfunctional endothelium $\downarrow$ NO, PGI$_2$, CD39 $\uparrow$ Endothelial permeability $\uparrow$ Adhesion molecules | Infiltration of monocytes and LDL cholesterol Generation of foam cells | Vulnerable plaque Thin fibrous cap with procoagulant, proinflammatory and prothrombotic plaque, susceptible to rupture, causing acute coronary occlusion |

Figure 1.4 Atherogenic plaque formation. The proatherogenic environment of dysfunctional endothelium allows transformation of monocytes to macrophages, which engulf LDL cholesterol particles to create foam cells and form fatty yellow streaks. The extracellular matrix that separates the plaque from the arterial lumen (fibrous cap) is weak and prone to rupture. LDL, low-density lipoprotein; NO, nitric oxide.

Plaque vulnerability

A vulnerable plaque is prone to rupture or erosion, leading to platelet-rich thrombosis generation and subsequently to ACS. Histologically, a vulnerable plaque consists of a thin-capped fibroatheroma that is enriched in cholesterol debris, a large number of inflammatory cells – especially macrophages, some activated T cells, and smooth muscle cells. Plaque vulnerability is influenced by a dynamic balance between collagen synthesis and degradation by MMPs. Together, the leukocytes and endothelial cells proliferate at the plaque site and secrete extracellular matrix components and MMPs that degrade collagen and cause plaque erosion (see below). Similarly, macrophages can also elicit apoptosis of the smooth muscle cells of the plaque that may further affect the collagen synthesis and ensure thinning of the fibrous cap. Large amounts of hyaluronan (an anionic non-sulfated glycosaminoglycan that is present in both eroded and ruptured plaques) promote thrombosis by enhancing local adherence of platelets and leukocytes.

Over the years, plaque volumes can markedly enlarge (positive remodeling) and thereby reduce the arterial lumen area below a critical point, resulting in ischemia and angina pectoris. However, even advanced atherosclerosis can remain clinically silent if arterial stenoses do not limit the blood flow. The downstream arterioles will dilate to compensate for the stenosis. The severity of flow obstruction depends on plaque size, vasoconstriction (spasm) and remodeling of the vessel wall. Symptoms only occur when oxygen demand exceeds the supply. Resting blood flow through a stenosed artery is not significantly affected until the luminal area is reduced by about 80% (or the diameter by at least 50%), although flow reserve is decreased at earlier stages of obstruction. The relationships between plaque morphology, arterial remodeling and stenosis formation are not consistent; many stenoses develop in a phasic rather than a linear manner, with high-grade stenoses forming at sites that were only insignificantly narrowed the year before.

Plaque rupture

Plaque rupture is more common among men (78%) than women (60%), and is less frequently observed in premenopausal women. The major determinants of thrombus generation are those of the classic 'triad of Virchow':

- thrombogenicity of the exposed plaque material (plaque vulnerability)
- local flow disturbances (vessel vulnerability)
- systemic thrombotic propensity (blood vulnerability).

Whatever the cause of endothelial denudation (plaque vulnerability), it may be a weaker thrombogenic stimulus, whereas flow disturbances (stasis, turbulence), platelet hyperreactivity, hypercoagulability, inflammation and depressed fibrinolysis (blood vulnerability) play major roles. In addition, atherosclerotic lesion development and thrombotic complications are confined to areas characterized by low shear rate and/or flow disturbances (e.g. narrow vessels, bifurcations and branching points) (Figure 1.5).

The underlying mechanisms of vulnerable plaque development (fibrous cap thinning and propensity to rupture) and thrombus generation at the site of plaque rupture are poorly understood. It is estimated that frank plaque rupture is responsible for about 75% of coronary thromboses, whereas endothelial erosion without frank plaque rupture, which is more common in women, accounts for 20%. Erosions around calcium nodules, rapid plaque expansion and intraplaque hemorrhage account for the remaining occurrences of

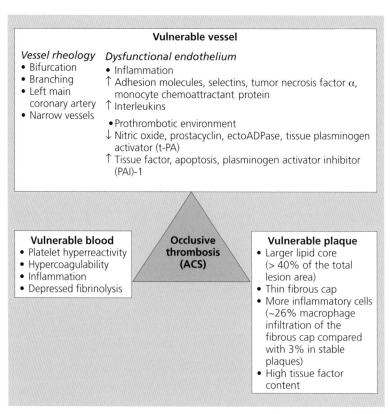

Figure 1.5 The 'triad of Virchow': contributors to thrombus formation.

thrombosis and vessel occlusions. It has been demonstrated that only a small percentage of plaque ruptures occur at sites of severe arterial stenoses, and in most cases high-grade coronary arterial stenoses are preceded by multiple healed plaque ruptures.

Distal microembolization. Microemboli of plaque material and thrombus may be washed downstream from the culprit lesion leading to distal microembolization, whereas iatrogenic embolization may occur during percutaneous coronary interventions (PCIs). Thus, distal emboli from either source may cause microvascular obstruction and myocardial ischemia/infarction despite a recanalized infarct-related epicardial coronary artery. In addition to thrombus generation at the culprit plaque rupture site, multiple plaque ruptures and luminal thrombi may occur in ACS patients. Moreover, the risk of new thrombus generation at the site of a non-culprit lesion is high during the 12 months after initial presentation in ACS patients.

Culprit lesions. Clinical studies utilizing angioscopy or intravascular ultrasound (IVUS) have demonstrated that on average less than 5% of lesions in patients at risk progress to culprit stage; subsequent ischemic events occur in equal proportions at regions that have or have not been the culprit lesion for the index event. Non-culprit lesions that were responsible for unanticipated subsequent thrombotic events were angiographically mild at the baseline and characterized by thin-cap fibroatheroma, large plaque burden ($\geq 70\%$) or small luminal area (≤ 4 mm^2). Lesions with a large necrotic core and thin fibrous cap, together known as thin-cap fibroatheroma, are highly predictive of progression to culprit lesions and are an independent risk factor for major cardiovascular events. Moreover, only occasionally (1%) a major life-threatening thrombus or acute coronary event develops at the site of a plaque rupture (Figure 1.6). Therefore, coronary event occurrence requires a 'perfect storm' in which numerous cardiovascular risk factors and classic Virchow's triad converge. These findings suggest that coronary disease is a dynamic and unpredictable process, and prediction of plaque vulnerability and ischemic event occurrence is still a mirage.

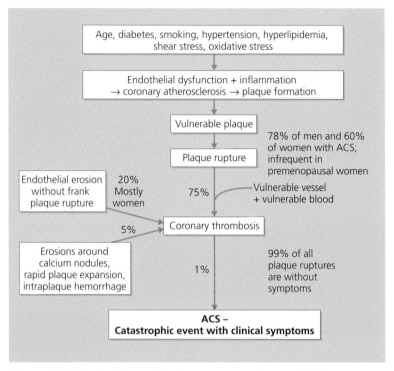

Figure 1.6 Pathophysiology of acute coronary syndromes (ACS).

Thrombus generation

Platelets play a central role in the genesis of thrombosis at the site of vessel wall injury (Figure 1.7). Atherosclerotic plaque rupture and endothelial denudation result in the exposure of the subendothelial matrix and the release of various factors such as cholesterol, tissue factor and necrotic debris. These factors facilitate platelet adhesion and activation. Under the high shear conditions present in arterial blood vessels, initial platelet adhesion is facilitated by binding of the glycoprotein (GP) Ib/IX/V receptor to von Willebrand factor (vWF) immobilized on collagen and binding of the GPVI receptor directly to exposed collagen.

Following adhesion, platelets form a monolayer at the site of vessel wall injury (primary hemostasis) and undergo activation. The activation process results in morphologic changes coupled with intracellular calcium ion mobilization resulting in the release of

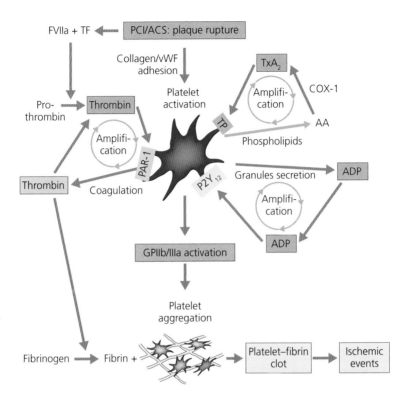

Figure 1.7 Mechanism of thrombus generation: plaque rupture releases factors that facilitate platelet adhesion and activation, and the release of secondary agonists (TxA_2 and ADP) sustains platelet aggregation. In addition, the release of tissue factor – following plaque rupture – generates thrombin, which in turn converts fibrinogen to fibrin, resulting in a stable occlusive platelet–fibrin clot. The amplification of thrombin generation on the surface of platelets is the major source of thrombin. AA, arachidonic acid; ACS, acute coronary syndrome; ADP, adenosine diphosphate; COX, cyclo-oxygenase; FVIIa, activated factor VII; GP, glycoprotein; PAR-1, platelet protease-activated receptor for thrombin; PCI, percutaneous intervention; $P2Y_{12}$, platelet receptor for ADP; TF, tissue factor; TP, platelet receptor for thromboxane; TxA_2, thromboxane A_2; vWF, von Willebrand factor.

procoagulant and proinflammatory microparticles and chemokines. The subsequent intracellular events, particularly downstream from GPVI, lead to the release of the important secondary agonists thromboxane (Tx) A_2 and adenosine diphosphate (ADP). TxA_2 is produced from membrane phospholipids, and ADP is released from dense granules. Through autocrine and paracrine mechanisms, these two locally generated secondary agonists play a critical role in sustaining platelet activation, and finally the activation of GPIIb/IIIa receptors (final common pathway).

Binding of activated GPIIb/IIIa receptors via fibrinogen molecules between adjacent platelets results in stable and robust thrombus generation at the site of vessel wall injury. It has been proposed that sustained platelet activation of the GPIIb/IIIa receptor and platelet procoagulant activity are critically dependent on continuous signaling downstream from the $P2Y_{12}$ receptor, an important ADP receptor.

Plaque rupture also results in tissue factor exposure at the site of vascular injury and the generation of small amounts of thrombin, the most potent primary platelet agonist. Thrombin further promotes platelet activation and the formation of a procoagulant platelet surface where larger amounts of thrombin are produced through the coagulation process.

Finally, thrombin converts fibrinogen to fibrin leading to the formation of an extensive fibrin network and a stable occlusive platelet–fibrin clot. In addition to the prothrombotic properties resulting from heightened platelet reactivity, a procoagulant and antifibrinolytic environment in the presence of a dysfunctional endothelium and plaque rupture markedly enhances clot formation and stability.

The clinical manifestation of thrombus generation at the site of plaque rupture depends on the extent and duration of thrombotic occlusion. Mural platelet-rich 'white' thrombi most often incompletely block coronary blood flow and are present in UA and NSTEMI. STEMI is often characterized by the complete obstruction of coronary vessels by 'red thrombi' rich in red blood cells and fibrin that overlay platelet-rich thrombi (see Figure 1.1). In contrast to UA/NSTEMI, STEMI more often results in abrupt and persistent ischemia which, if left untreated, can cause sudden cardiac death.

Key points – pathophysiology

- The common underlying mechanism of acute coronary syndromes (ACS) is atherosclerotic plaque rupture or erosion, with differing degrees of superimposed thrombosis and distal embolization.
- Although atherosclerosis starts with the development of dysfunctional endothelium in the presence of cardiovascular risk factors early in life, the speed of progression is non-linear, unpredictable and varies markedly between individuals.
- A vulnerable plaque is prone to rupture or erosion and consists of a thin-capped fibroatheroma that is enriched in cholesterol debris, a large number of inflammatory cells (especially macrophages, some activated T cells), and smooth muscle cells.
- The major determinants of thrombus generation are those of the classic 'triad of Virchow': thrombogenicity of the exposed plaque material (plaque vulnerability), local flow disturbances (vessel vulnerability), and systemic thrombotic propensity (blood vulnerability).
- Mural platelet-rich 'white' thrombi most often incompletely block coronary blood flow and are present in unstable angina (UA) and non-ST-segment elevation myocardial infarction (NSTEMI).
- ST-segment elevation MI (STEMI) is often characterized by the complete obstruction of coronary vessels by thrombi rich in red blood cells and fibrin, which overlay platelet-rich thrombi.

Key references

Naghavi M, Libby P, Falk E et al. From vulnerable plaque to vulnerable patient: a call for new definitions and risk assessment strategies: Part II. *Circulation* 2003;108:1772–8.

Stone GW, Maehara A, Lansky AJ et al.; PROSPECT Investigators. A prospective natural-history study of coronary atherosclerosis. *N Engl J Med* 2011;364:226–35.

Wright RS, Anderson JL, Adams CD et al. 2011 ACCF/AHA focused update incorporated into the ACC/AHA 2007 Guidelines for the Management of Patients with Unstable Angina/Non-ST-Elevation Myocardial Infarction: a report of the American College of Cardiology Foundation/American Heart Association Task Force on Practice Guidelines developed in collaboration with the American Academy of Family Physicians, Society for Cardiovascular Angiography and Interventions, and the Society of Thoracic Surgeons. *J Am Coll Cardiol* 2011;57:e215–367.

2 Diagnosis, risk stratification and decision-making

Acute coronary syndromes (ACS) occur in a heterogeneous patient population who present with various clinical symptoms ranging from atypical to typical chest discomfort. Accompanying ECG changes can be non-specific, or involve ST-segment elevation or depression. At presentation, cardiac biomarkers may be normal or elevated. Outside of clinical trials, the overall mortality rate in the first month in patients with myocardial infarction (MI) or ACS is estimated at 15–30%; most of these deaths occur within 2 hours of the MI. In recent randomized large-scale trials, the 30-day in-hospital mortality rate was 4–10%, 7–10% in patients qualified for fibrinolysis and 4–6% in those qualified for fibrinolysis and/or coronary interventions. Mortality is higher in the registries, indicating that patients included in randomized studies are at a lower risk than individuals in the 'real world'.

In this scenario, the keys to optimizing patient outcomes in ACS are:
- accurate initial diagnosis
- appropriate risk stratification
- proper therapeutic decision-making.

Clinical recognition of ACS requires a careful assessment of the clinical presentation and history, application of appropriate imaging techniques and measurement of biomarkers.

Clinical presentation and history

The most important factors to consider when taking the patient's history are the nature of the angina symptoms (see below), a history of coronary artery disease (CAD) (in up to 80% of patients), male gender, older age and a number of traditional cardiovascular risk factors such as smoking, family history, hyperlipidemia, diabetes and hypertension. These last traditional risk factors are poor predictors of the likelihood of ACS, but they may be associated with poorer outcomes.

Chest pain. The hallmark symptom of ACS is pain in the center (substernal) or left of the chest, with radiation to the left shoulder and arm, neck and jaw (Table 2.1); pain in the arm is usually on the inner (ulnar) aspect. Most often, pain in the chest feels like a pressure or heaviness lasting for more than 20 minutes. It may or may not be severe. Chest pain in the setting of ST-segment elevation myocardial infarction (STEMI) usually occurs at rest, while in the setting of unstable angina/non-ST-segment elevation MI (UA/NSTEMI) chest pain often occurs during activity and stops at rest.

Less commonly, patients may present with epigastric pain, which is frequently mistaken for indigestion. Occasionally, chest pain may be perceived in the right side of the chest or intrascapular region. Severe pain that radiates through the chest into the back is more suggestive of aortic dissection than ACS. Pain that the patient can localize by pointing with one finger, or that worsens after pressing the chest, is infrequently ischemic in origin (ischemic pain usually occupies a substantially large area). The Levine sign, in which a patient places a clenched fist over the chest while describing the pain, is classically seen in patients with MI.

Useful questions to ask the patient about their chest pain include:
- What does it feel like?
- Where is it located?
- Does it stay in one spot or does it radiate to another spot?
- When do you notice it? What brings it on?
- Is it associated with exertion, meals or certain body positions?
- How long does it last?
- How severe is it?
- When was the last episode?
- Have you found anything that makes it feel better?
- Have you found anything that makes it feel worse?
- Can you reproduce it by pushing on your chest wall?

Physical examination

A symptom-oriented physical examination should be performed to identify any consequences of acute ischemia and resultant cardiac dysfunction, and to rule out non-cardiac causes of chest pain such as non-ischemic cardiovascular disorders (e.g. pulmonary embolism,

TABLE 2.1

Symptoms of acute coronary syndromes

Pain or discomfort
- Substernal, upper abdominal or epigastric
- Radiating to neck, jaw, shoulders, back and/or one or both arms

- Described as sensation of pressure, crushing, tightness, heaviness, cramping, burning, aching
- Accompanying dyspnea, indigestion, nausea, vomiting, diaphoresis
- Associated hypotension or ventricular arrhythmias

Other typical symptoms
- Isolated dyspnea
- Weakness
- Diaphoresis
- Light-headedness and/or syncope
- Nausea and vomiting

Atypical symptoms
- Palpitations
- Anxiety
- Sense of impending doom
- No typical chest pain/'anginal equivalents' (angina symptoms at sites other than the chest or other complaints like dyspnea only)*

Symptoms of clinical instability
- Progressive angina (new-onset angina with progressive symptoms, or more frequent, severe or prolonged pain than previously, triggered at a lower exercise threshold or at rest)
- Prolonged chest pain (≥ 20 minutes)

*Most likely in the elderly, women and individuals with diabetes (~ 30% of ACS patients). These individuals are 2.2 times more likely to die during hospitalization than those with typical symptoms.
Adapted from Fitchett DH et al. 2011.

aortic dissection, pericarditis, valvular heart disease) and pulmonary diseases. Physical signs that may be helpful in differentiating non-ischemic from ischemic etiologies of chest pain are shown in Table 2.2.

The physical examination should include an assessment of vital signs, jugular venous pressure, heart sounds and murmurs, and peripheral perfusion. Auscultation of the chest may provide evidence of congestive heart failure. The abdomen should also be examined (a palpable abdominal mass indicates aortic aneurysm) and skin color assessed. The neurological examination should focus on the level of patient alertness and any evidence of stroke.

Patients with ACS frequently exhibit anxiety and restlessness, diaphoresis and skin pallor. The patient may have a variable heart rate, depending on the degree of anxiety, concomitant arrhythmias and hemodynamic compromise. Body temperature is likely to be normal in patients with UA but elevated during MI. Respiratory rate may be normal or elevated because of pain, anxiety or left ventricular (LV) dysfunction. An abnormal cardiac examination will be observed more often in patients with MI than in those with UA.

TABLE 2.2

Physical signs of non-ischemic chest pain

Physical sign	Likely cause
Reproduction of pain on palpation	Musculoskeletal problem
Difference in blood pressure between the upper and lower limbs	Aortic dissection
Irregular pulse	Atrial fibrillation
Specific heart murmurs	Aortic stenosis or aortic insufficiency secondary to an ascending aortic dissecting aneurysm
Pericardial or pleural friction rub	Pericarditis or pleuritis, respectively
Abdominal mass	Aortic aneurysm

Electrocardiography

A resting 12-lead ECG should be performed and reviewed by an experienced clinician in all patients with suspected ACS within 10 minutes of first medical contact. If the likelihood of ACS is high but the 12-lead ECG is normal, a 17-lead ECG may be performed to reveal 'true posterior' STEMI (usually caused by occlusion of the circumflex artery or upper marginal branch of the circumflex artery). Without this, 8–10% of STEMIs may be misdiagnosed as NSTEMIs.

Since ECGs provide only a 'snap shot' of myocardial ischemia, continuous monitoring and serial ECG tracings are recommended. Continuous monitoring provides vital information about arrhythmias or the development of recurrent ischemia. European (ESC) guidelines recommend that an ECG should be recorded at least 6 and 24 hours after presentation and if/when symptoms recur. It is important to compare current and previous ECG findings, as patients with no ECG changes have a lower risk of complications than those with ECG changes.

ST-segment deviation. New ST-segment deviation, even of 0.05 mV, is an important and specific measure of ischemia and prognosis.

ST-segment depression of 0.05 mV or more in two or more contiguous leads, in the appropriate clinical context, is suggestive of non-ST-elevation ACS (NSTEMI and UA). Minor ST-segment depression (< 0.05 mV) may be difficult to interpret. ST-segment depression of 0.1 mV or greater is more clinically relevant and is associated with an 11% rate of death and MI at 1 year. ST-segment depression of 0.2 mV or more carries about a sixfold increased mortality risk. ST-segment depression combined with transient ST elevation identifies an even higher-risk subgroup.

ST-segment elevation of 0.1 mV or more in at least two contiguous leads indicates acute MI in 90% of patients. Persistent ST elevation for more than 20 minutes suggests STEMI (see Figure 1.1). A new left bundle branch block (LBBB) is indicative of STEMI; a new right bundle branch block (RBBB) may also be associated with acute STEMI.

Close monitoring of the degree of ST-segment elevation after fibrinolysis provides a non-invasive method of assessing reperfusion (see Chapter 5). The degree of ST-segment elevation resolution after reperfusion therapy has been associated with both short- and long-term outcomes.

25

T-wave inversion is sensitive for ischemia but is less specific, unless it is marked ($\geq$ 0.3 mV).

Other tests, although not usually performed on a routine basis, may help to identify patients at greatest risk of arrhythmic death. The definitive roles of these novel techniques require further evaluation in large-scale trials.

An 80-lead ECG (such as the PRIME ECG) can analyze a 360-degree spatial view of the heart. It can improve the rapid and accurate diagnosis of STEMI, particularly ischemia in the high right anterior, posterior and right ventricular territories.

Heart rate variability, measured by 24-hour Holter monitoring, is the standard deviation of normal to normal RR interval (SDNN). When added to baroreceptor reflex sensitivity (a marker of the body's ability to reflexively increase vagal activity and decrease sympathetic activity in response to a sudden increase in blood pressure), SDNN improves the discrimination of risk of death after MI.

Deceleration capacity. In this technique, a signal processing algorithm separately characterizes deceleration and acceleration of heart rate to distinguish between vagal and sympathetic factors that affect heart rate variability. Risk stratification based on deceleration capacity is significantly better than measurement of left ventricular ejection fraction (LVEF) and SDNN, and substantially improves risk prediction in survivors of acute MI.

Heart rate turbulence is a measure of the short-term fluctuations in sinus cycle length after premature ventricular contractions, i.e. a brief speeding up of heart rate followed by a slow decrease back to the baseline rate. It reflects minute hemodynamic disturbances that occur after premature ventricular beats, and is one of the strongest independent post-MI risk predictors.

T-wave alternans is measured during bicycle exercise stress testing. Using noise reduction signal processing enables microvolt electrical alternans of the T wave ('microscopic' TWA) to be detected, which may be associated with an increased risk of ventricular arrhythmias in several clinical settings.

Markers of myocardial injury

Prolonged reductions in blood flow result in myocardial necrosis and the release of cardiac-specific enzymes and other substances into the circulation (Table 2.3). Elevated circulating levels of these substances

TABLE 2.3

Markers of myocardial injury

	Biomarker	Advantages
Myocardial necrosis	Cardiac troponins	Facilitate the diagnosis, prognosis and clinical implication of ACS/MI
Endogenous stress	Copeptin	Rules out ACS
Inflammation	C-reactive protein, myeloperoxidase, pregnancy-associated protein, ST2 (a member of the interleukin 1 receptor family)	Indicate inflammation during ACS
Ventricular stress	BNP, NT-proBNP	Facilitate prognosis and clinical implication
Thrombosis	Platelet aggregation, single nucleotide polymorphisms of cytochrome genes, soluble CD40 ligand, P-selectin, D-dimer, vWF, fibrinogen, PAI-1, t-PA	Indicate antiplatelet drug response, a prothrombotic mileu and clinical implication
Ischemia	Ischemia-modified albumin, heart fatty acid binding protein, growth differentiating factor-15	Help in the prognosis of the disease
Cholesterol/ lipoprotein metabolism	Lysosomal phospholipase A2	

ACS, acute coronary syndromes; BNP, B-type natriuretic peptide; MI, myocardial infarction; NT-proBNP, N-terminal prohormone fragment of BNP; PAI-1, plasminogen activator inhibitor-1; t-PA, tissue plasminogen activator; vWF, von Willebrand factor.
Adapted from Scirica BM 2010.

are a hallmark of MI. Since ACS and the development of ischemic events following ACS are influenced by numerous pathophysiological pathways, a multimarker approach may improve risk stratification.

Cardiac troponins I and T are specific for myocardial injury, highly sensitive in detecting small amounts of myocardial necrosis, and the preferred markers for the diagnosis of MI. Cardiac troponins are also markers of active thrombogenic plaque, detecting microscopic infarctions, which may be due to severe ischemia and/or distal microembolization of unstable plaque contents (platelet-platelet aggregates, platelet-leukocyte aggregates, atherosclerotic debris). They are therefore a useful indicator in patients at high risk of ACS and are helpful in guiding therapies. Troponins can be detected in blood samples as early as 2–4 hours after the onset of myocardial necrosis and remain elevated for up to 5–14 days (Figure 2.1).

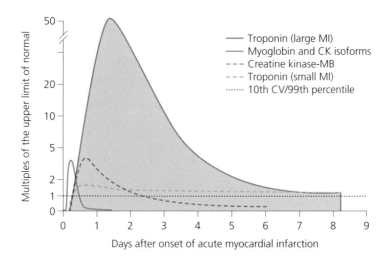

Figure 2.1 Timing of release of various biomarkers after acute myocardial infarction (MI). Adapted from Shapiro BP, Jaffe AS. Cardiac biomarkers. In: Murphy JG, Lloyd MA, eds. *Mayo Clinic Cardiology: Concise Textbook*, 3rd ed. Rochester, MN: Mayo Clinic Scientific Press and New York: Informa Healthcare USA, 2007:773–80.

Cardiac troponins as prognostic indicators. Troponin values above the 99th percentile of a normal population are considered to be elevated and an indicator of myocardial necrosis. Overall, an elevated troponin level is associated with a fourfold increase in risk of death or recurrent MI compared with a normal troponin concentration. However, cardiac troponin levels should be considered in conjunction with other risk factors such as age, renal function and ECG changes. In STEMI patients, elevated troponin on admission is associated with worse outcomes, and peak troponin concentrations correlate with infarct size determined by nuclear imaging. Elevated troponin levels reflect severe ischemia associated with necrosis that is typically due to more complex and thrombotic lesions. Therefore, patients with elevated troponin derive the greatest benefit from aggressive antithrombotic therapies.

New high-sensitivity troponin assays detect pg/mL to ng/mL levels of troponin and offer greater sensitivity and earlier detection of very low levels of myocardial injury than older assays; however, they may be associated with reduced specificity. Treatment strategies based on older troponin assays, including early invasive management, may now require reassessment as more sensitive assays are available in clinical practice.

Other cardiac biomarkers. Creatine kinase-MB (CK-MB) is less specific and less sensitive than cardiac troponins but may be useful in the detection of early reinfarction. Myoglobin has very low specificity but high sensitivity and is useful in the early detection of MI. A comparison of the advantages and disadvantages of cardiac markers is given in Table 2.4.

Other biomarkers. In addition to the cardiac markers discussed above, markers of inflammation, platelet activation and neurohormonal activation have been used in the diagnosis and risk stratification of ACS.

Markers of inflammation. C-reactive protein (CRP) is hepatically synthesized in response to inflammatory signals, is found in atherosclerotic plaques and has been reported to contribute to plaque instability. High-sensitivity CRP (hsCRP) has been associated with the

29

TABLE 2.4

Cardiac biomarkers in patients with suspected acute coronary syndromes but no ST-segment elevation

Marker	Advantages	Disadvantages
Cardiac troponins	• Powerful tool for risk stratification • Greater sensitivity and specificity than CK-MB • Detection of recent MI up to 2 weeks after onset • Useful for selection of therapy • Detection of reperfusion	• Low sensitivity in early phase of MI (< 6 hours after symptom onset); requires repeat measurement at 8–12 hours if negative • Limited ability to detect late minor reinfarction
CK-MB	• Rapid, cost-efficient, accurate assays • Ability to detect early reinfarction	• Loss of specificity in patients with skeletal muscle disease or injury, including surgery • Low sensitivity during early MI (< 6 hours after symptom onset) or later (> 36 hours after symptom onset) and for minor myocardial damage (detectable with troponins)
Myoglobin	• High sensitivity • Useful in early detection of MI • Detection of reperfusion • Most useful in ruling out MI	• Very low specificity in patients with skeletal muscle injury or disease • Rapid return to normal range limits, reducing sensitivity for later presentations

CK-MB, MB fraction of creatine kinase; MI, myocardial infarction.

risk of coronary heart disease in a generally healthy population (odds ratio 1.45), and has been independently associated with short- and long-term patient risk in NSTEMI and STEMI. In most studies, hsCRP greater than 3 mg/L was associated with cardiovascular risk. Compared with admission levels of hsCRP, discharge levels of hsCRP have been shown to be more predictive of death, MI and recurrent ischemia at 1 year. However, the diagnostic value of hsCRP in ACS has not been firmly established. The timing of CRP measurement is critical, since CRP levels may change between ACS presentation and recovery. Other markers of inflammation are shown in Table 2.3.

Markers of neurohormonal activation. The natriuretic peptides B-type natriuretic peptide (BNP) and the N-terminal prohormone fragment (NT-proBNP) are released from the ventricular myocardium by hypoxia, ischemia, increased wall stress, and ventricular and atrial dilation. Both are powerful predictors of death and recurrent MI in NSTEMI and STEMI, independent of troponin and CRP levels. BNP and NT-proBNP are useful markers in the emergency room in differentiating cardiac and non-cardiac causes of dyspnea with age-dependent cutoffs. In addition to elevated levels during heart failure, these markers are elevated during pulmonary hypertension, pulmonary embolism, cardiac arrhythmia, cardiac ischemia and aortic stenosis. Therefore, these markers lack specificity to either include or exclude patients with ACS.

Natriuretic peptide levels usually increase after the initiation of ACS, with peak levels observed hours after the ACS episode, gradually decreasing days later. Persistently elevated levels in the days and weeks after an ACS episode may identify patients with a high risk for cardiovascular death or heart failure, even in the setting of a normal ejection fraction. Although these markers appear useful for long-term prognosis, their usefulness for initial risk stratification is limited. Moreover, the optimal time to measure BNP and the definitive cutoff value for prognosis have not yet been defined.

Markers of acute endogenous stress. Copeptin, also called c-terminal pro-vasopressin, is a new marker that is co-secreted with vasopressin from the hypothalamus in response to the changes in plasma osmolarity and arterial hypovolemia. Copeptin levels rise to their maximum immediately after symptom onset and decrease below the cut-off within 10 hours. In contrast to conventional cardiac biomarkers that reach their peak levels 14–16 hours after the onset of symptoms, a rapid increase in copeptin levels following ACS may help in faster diagnosis and treatment of ACS patients.

Coagulation or endogenous fibrinolysis markers such as fibrinogen, prothrombin fragments, fibrinopeptide and D-dimer, as well as plasminogen activator-inhibitor-1 (PAI-1) or tissue plasminogen activator (t-PA) are elevated during ACS, but have limited specificity and diagnostic utility. Measurements of platelet reactivity are gaining more importance as cardiovascular risk factors in patients treated with percutaneous coronary interventions. However, their usefulness in deciding optimal treatment strategies associated with improved outcomes has not been demonstrated (see below).

Markers of impaired renal function, which is a strong predictor of long-term mortality in ACS patients, include creatinine clearance or glomerular filtration rate. However, because these measurements are affected by age, weight, race and various medications, their value as an independent risk marker for ACS patients is limited.

Definition of myocardial infarction

An international task force recently defined the type of MI according to the circumstances that cause it (i.e. spontaneous or in the setting of a diagnostic or therapeutic procedure), the amount of cell loss (infarct size) and the timing of the MI (i.e. evolving, healing or healed) (Table 2.5).

In addition, either one of the following criteria satisfy the diagnosis of an acute, evolving or recent MI:

- A typical rise and gradual fall in troponin levels, or a more rapid rise and fall in CK-MB levels, plus at least one of:
  - ischemic symptoms
  - development of pathological Q waves on the ECG
  - ECG changes indicative of ischemia (ST-segment elevation or depression)
  - coronary artery intervention (e.g. coronary angioplasty).
- Pathological findings of an acute MI.

TABLE 2.5

Classification of myocardial infarction

Type 1: Spontaneous MI

- Atherosclerotic plaque rupture, ulceration, fissuring, erosion or dissection
- Intraluminal thrombus in ≥ 1 coronary artery
- Decreased myocardial blood flow or distal platelet emboli with ensuing myocyte necrosis
- Underlying severe CAD or, on occasion, non-obstructive or no CAD

Type 2: MI secondary to ischemic imbalance

- Myocardial injury with necrosis
- Condition other than CAD contributes to imbalance between myocardial oxygen supply and/or demand:
  - coronary endothelial dysfunction
  - coronary artery spasm
  - coronary embolism
  - tachy- or bradyarrhythmias
  - anemia
  - respiratory failure
  - hypotension
  - hypertension with or without LVH

Type 3: MI resulting in death; no biomarker values available

- Cardiac death with symptoms suggestive of myocardial ischemia
- Presumed new ischemic ECG changes or new LBBB
- Death occurs before blood samples obtained or cardiac biomarkers rise, or in rare cases cardiac biomarkers are not collected

CONTINUED

TABLE 2.5 (CONTINUED)

Type 4a: MI related to PCI

- Elevated cTn values > 5 times the 99th percentile URL,* or > 20% rise above elevated baseline values, stable or falling
- Also, one of:
  - symptoms suggestive of myocardial ischemia
  - new ischemic ECG changes or new LBBB
  - angiographic loss of patency of major coronary artery or side branch, or persistent slow or no flow or embolization
  - imaging evidence of new loss of viable myocardium or new regional wall motion abnormality

Type 4b: MI related to stent thrombosis

- Detected by coronary angiography or autopsy in the setting of myocardial ischemia
- Rise and/ or fall of cardiac biomarkers with ≥ 1 value above the 99th percentile URL*

Type 5: MI related to CABG

- Elevated cardiac biomarker values > 10 times the 99th percentile URL*
- Also, one of:
  - new pathological Q waves or new LBBB
  - angiographic documented new graft or new native coronary artery occlusion
  - imaging evidence of new loss of viable myocardium or new regional wall motion abnormality.

*In patients with normal baseline values (≤ 99th percentile URL).
CABG, coronary artery bypass grafting; CAD, coronary artery disease; cTn, cardiac troponin; LBBB, left bundle branch block; LVH, left ventricular hypertrophy; MI, myocardial infarction; PCI, percutaneous coronary intervention; URL, upper reference limit.
Adapted from Thygesen K et al., 2012

Any one of the following criteria satisfies the diagnosis of an established or previous MI:

- Development of new pathological Q waves on serial ECGs. The patient may or may not remember previous symptoms. Biochemical markers of myocardial necrosis may have normalized, depending on the length of time that has passed since the infarct developed.
- Imaging evidence of a region of loss of viable myocardium that is thinned and fails to contract in the absence of a non-ischemic cause.
- Pathological findings of a healed or healing MI.

Imaging

In the future, non-invasive cardiac imaging may play a major role in the diagnosis of ACS. At present, its clinical utility is greatest in patients with an intermediate probability of ACS. Echocardiography may help to identify ischemic regions by detecting new wall motion abnormalities. In patients with a high probability of ACS (typical symptoms, documented CAD, elevated cardiac biomarker levels, dynamic ECG changes) non-invasive imaging will not offer much incremental clinical information, whereas in patients with a very low probability of ACS further imaging may only increase the chance of false-positive results.

Imaging techniques can determine ventricular function or the coronary anatomy responsible for ACS. In patients with ongoing chest discomfort but non-diagnostic ECG and biomarkers, active ischemia can be identified by resting myocardial perfusion imaging (MPI). MPI will not distinguish recent and old infarcts, but MPI with single-photon emission computed tomography (SPECT) and contrast echocardiography can identify areas of recent ischemia and may improve early diagnosis of ACS. Cardiac magnetic resonance (CMR) imaging can define ventricular function, identify ongoing ischemia and reperfusion, and distinguish old and young infarcts; coronary anatomy can also be determined.

Invasive coronary angiography is the primary tool to identify significant lesions that require intervention. However, CT angiography (CTA) provides excellent resolution of the coronary anatomy. Echocardiography is the most commonly used technique to assess ventricular function and complications of MI; however, SPECT and CMR imaging provide substantial information regarding infarct size and left ventricular function.

Ischemic risk stratification

Numerous risk stratification algorithms and scores have been developed in patients with ACS, based on the results of large clinical trials and registries, and have been validated independently in large cohort studies. These include the Thrombolysis in Myocardial Infarction (TIMI) score, Global Registry of Acute Coronary Events (GRACE), Platelet glycoprotein IIb/IIIa in Unstable angina: Receptor Suppression Using Integrilin Therapy (PURSUIT) score and Controlled Abciximab and Device Investigation to Lower Late Angioplasty Complications (CADILLAC) score.

The TIMI score is based on seven independent, easily assessed prognostic variables. Patients with three or more of the seven variables are considered to be at greater risk of a composite endpoint of all-cause mortality, MI and severe recurrent ischemia, prompting urgent revascularization after 14 days. Those with no more than two variables are considered to be at low risk (Table 2.6).

The GRACE risk score. In the GRACE risk model, eight variables are used to predict whether a patient will die or have a MI in the hospital or in the next 6 months. Each variable is assigned a numeric score on the basis of a specific value, and the eight scores are added to yield a total score, which is applied to a reference nomogram to determine the patient's risk (www.outcomes-umassmed.org/grace/acs_risk/acs_risk_content.html, last accessed 04 November 2013). GRACE uses variables derived from a registry of consecutive ACS patients, rather than patients in randomized trials (as in other scores) with specific inclusion-exclusion criteria. GRACE also includes renal function as a variable, since this is known to influence long-term prognosis.

Application of risk scores. Ischemic risk scores assist risk stratification at the time of hospital admission, help to identify patients suitable for early invasive management and predict short- and long-term adverse cardiac events. Table 2.7 shows predicted in-hospital and short-term (14-day), as well as long-term (6-month), outcomes in patients with ACS using the TIMI risk score and GRACE.

TABLE 2.6

The TIMI risk score for unstable angina/non-ST elevation MI

Variable	Score
Age ≥ 65 years	1
≥ 3 risk factors for CAD:	1
– Diabetes mellitus	
– Cigarette smoking	
– Hypertension (BP ≥ 140/90 mmHg or on hypertensive medication)	
– Low HDL cholesterol (< 40 mg/dL)	
– Family history of premature CAD	
ASA use in the last 7 days before hospitalization	1
Known CAD (stenosis ≥ 50%)	1
≥ 2 episodes of severe angina within 24 hours of hospitalization	1
ST-segment deviation (≥ 0.5 mm)	1
Positive cardiac markers (see text)	1

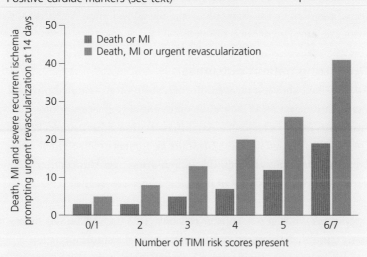

ASA, acetylsalicylic acid (aspirin); BP, blood pressure; CAD, coronary artery disease; HDL, high-density lipoprotein.
Adapted from Antman EM et al. 2000.

TABLE 2.7

Application of GRACE and TIMI risk scores to short- and long-term risk

	GRACE In-hospital	TIMI 14 days	GRACE 6 months
Low risk			
Score	≤ 108	0–2	≤ 88
Mortality	< 1%	1.1%	< 3%
Intermediate risk			
Score	109–140	3–4	89–118
Mortality	1–3%	2%	3–8%
High risk			
Score	≥ 140	5–7	≥ 118
Mortality	> 3%	5.8%	> 8%

International guidelines. The American College of Cardiology/ American Heart Association (ACC/AHA) have provided recommendations for establishing the likelihood of an ACS diagnosis from the initial evaluation (Table 2.8)

Optimizing patient outcomes

As described above, a targeted history, a symptom-oriented physical examination and an ECG are the main initial evaluation tools (see pages 21–6). The key initial differentiation is between STEMI and UA/NSTEMI based on the 12-lead ECG. Patients with STEMI require immediate therapies to establish infarct artery reperfusion that will depend on the availability of immediate invasive treatment (see Chapter 5, pages 88–98). As a clinical syndrome, ischemic discomfort without ST-segment elevation (UA and NSTEMI) shares some clinical characteristics with severe chronic stable angina, a condition associated with lower immediate risk.

Patients with hemodynamic compromise require immediate cardiac catheterization and revascularization with the potential for circulatory support. The timing of catheterization in the hemodynamically stable

TABLE 2.8

Likelihood that signs and symptoms indicate an acute coronary syndrome secondary to coronary artery disease

High likelihood *Any of the following:*	Intermediate likelihood *Absence of high-likelihood features and presence of any of the following:*	Low likelihood *Absence of high- or intermediate-likelihood features but may have:*
Pre-existing risk factors for atherosclerosis*		
≥ 3	1–2	0–1
History		
• Chest or left arm pain or discomfort as chief symptom, reproducing previously documented symptom • Angina • Known history of CAD, including MI	• Chest or left arm pain or discomfort as chief symptom • Age ≥ 70 years • Male gender • Diabetes mellitus	• Probable ischemic symptoms in the absence of any intermediate-likelihood characteristics • Recent cocaine use
Examination		
• Transient MR murmur • Hypotension • Diaphoresis • Pulmonary edema • Rales	• Extracardiac vascular disease	• Chest discomfort reproduced by palpation
ECG		
• New, or presumably new, transient ST-segment deviation (≥ 1 mm) • T-wave inversion in multiple precordial leads	• Fixed Q waves • ST depression 0.5–1.0 mm • T-wave inversion >1.0 mm	• T-wave flattening or inversion < 1 mm in leads with dominant R waves • Normal ECG tracing
Cardiac markers		
• Elevated cardiac TnI, TnT or CK-MB levels	• Normal	• Normal

CAD, coronary artery disease; CK-MB, muscle and brain fraction of creatine kinase; ECG, electrocardiogram; MI, myocardial infarction; MR, mitral regurgitation; TnI, troponin I; TnT, troponin T.
*Current smoking, hypertension, hyperlipidemia, diabetes mellitus, metabolic syndrome, positive family history (see also Table 1.1, page 10).

patient with UA/NSTEMI depends upon the assessment of risk. Therefore, proper initial diagnosis and risk stratification are critical to optimize patient outcomes in ACS (Figure 2.2).

Bleeding risk

Invasive and non-invasive management strategies for ACS reduce the recurrence of ischemic events, but are associated with an increased risk of bleeding. Importantly, major bleeding and the need for transfusion are associated with an increased risk of in-hospital mortality as well as a long-term risk of death or MI. Gastrointestinal and femoral access site bleeding during coronary angiography are the most frequent bleeding complications.

A variety of definitions for 'major' and 'minor' bleeding have been used in published clinical studies. In general, however, major bleeds can be considered those that are fatal or life-threatening, cause severe symptoms in a critical area or organ (e.g. intracranial, intraocular, intra-articular) or consume major healthcare resources. The International Society on Thrombosis and Haemostasis also gives a fall in hemoglobin level of 2.0 g/L (1.24 mmol/L) or more, or the need for transfusion of two or more units of whole or red blood cells, as a guideline for major bleeding in non-surgical patients. Minor bleeding can be considered any bleeding that requires medical intervention but does not cause hemodynamic compromise or require transfusion.

Clinical and therapeutic factors associated with an increased bleeding risk are shown in Table 2.9. Many of the characteristics associated with a heightened risk of bleeding are the same for ischemia.

Bleeding risk scores. The CRUSADE bleeding score was developed from the CRUSADE (Can Rapid risk stratification of Unstable angina patients Suppress ADverse outcomes with Early implementation of the ACC/AHA guidelines) registry and was further validated in a cohort of patients from the same registry. The score is divided into: very low risk (≤ 20); low risk (21–30); moderate risk (31–40); high risk (41–50); and very high risk (> 50). It has relatively high accuracy for estimating bleeding risk by incorporating admission and treatment variables (Table 2.10).

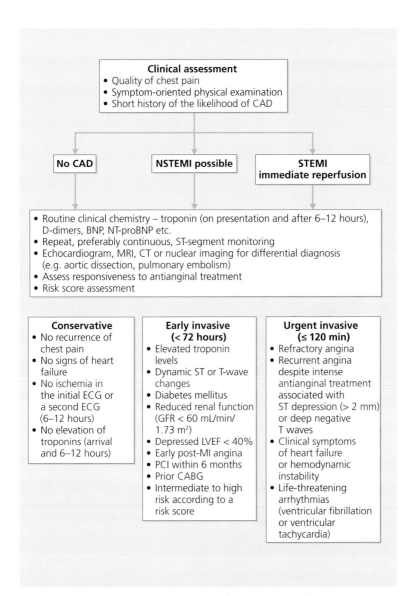

Figure 2.2 Early evaluation and risk stratification to optimize patient outcomes. BNP, B-type natriuretic peptide; CABG, coronary artery bypass grafting; CAD, coronary artery disease; GFR, glomerular filtration rate; LVEF, left ventricular ejection fraction; NSTEMI, non-ST-segment elevation MI; NT-proBNP, N-terminal prohormone fragment; PCI, percutaneous coronary intervention; STEMI, ST-segment elevation MI.

TABLE 2.9

Risk factors for bleeding

Clinical factors

- Advanced age[†]
- Female gender*[†]
- Low bodyweight
- History of bleeding
- Hypertension*
- Hemodynamic instability
- Increased risk of ischemic event (current heart failure or previous stroke, vascular disease or diabetes)*
- Anemia*[†]
- Hematocrit < 36%*[†]
- Renal insufficiency*[†]
- Creatinine clearance (increased risk per 10 mL/min decrease)*[†]
- Heart rate (increased risk per 10 bpm increase)*
- Elevated white blood cell count[†]
- Diagnosis of MI rather than UA[†]

Therapeutic factors

- Use of glycoprotein IIb/IIIa inhibitors
- Catheterization/PCI especially in first 24 hours
- Femoral access site
- Antiplatelet and/or antithrombotic overdosing
- Triple antithrombotic therapy (ASA, clopidogrel, and warfarin or other combinations)

*Variable associated with bleeding in the CRUSADE (Can Rapid Risk Stratification of Unstable Angina Patients Suppress Adverse Outcomes with Early Implementation of the ACC/AHA Guidelines) registry.
[†]Variable associated with major bleeding in the ACUITY (Acute Catheterization and Urgent Intervention Triage Strategy) and HORIZONS-AMI (Harmonizing Outcomes with Revascularization and Stents in Acute Myocardial Infarction) trials.
ASA, acetylsalicylic acid (aspirin); bpm, beats per minute; PCI, percutaneous coronary intervention.
Adapted from Fitchett DH et al. 2011.

The ACUITY bleeding risk score, derived from a pooled cohort of patients with ACS recruited in the Acute Catheterization and Urgent Intervention Triage strategy (ACUITY) and Harmonizing Outcomes

TABLE 2.10

CRUSADE risk score for in-hospital major bleeding

Predictor	Score	Predictor	Score
Baseline hematocrit (%)		Gender	
< 31	9	Male	0
31–33.9	7	Female	8
34–36.9	3	Signs of chronic heart failure at presentation	
37–39.9	2		
≥ 40	0		
		No	0
Creatinine clearance (mL/min)		Yes	7
≤ 15	39	Prior vascular disease	
> 15–30	35		
> 30–60	28	No	0
> 60–90	17	Yes	6
> 90–120	7	Diabetes mellitus	
> 120	0	No	0
		Yes	6
Heart rate (bpm)		Systolic BP (mmHg)	
≤ 70	0	≤ 90	10
71–80	1	91–100	8
81–90	3	101–120	5
91–100	6	121–180	1
101–110	8	181–200	3
111–120	10	≥ 201	5
≥ 121	11		

BP, blood pressure; bpm, beats per minute.
Total score: ≤ 20, very low risk; 21–30, low risk; 31–40, moderate risk; 41–50, high risk; > 50, very high risk.

with RevasculariZatiON and Stents in acute myocardial infarction (HORIZONS) trials, has been developed but not validated in an independent cohort. It is based on six independent baseline predictors (female gender, advanced age, elevated serum creatinine, white blood cell count, anemia, and NSTEMI or STEMI) and one treatment-related variable (use of heparin and a glycoprotein [GP] IIb/IIIa receptor inhibitor rather than bivalirudin alone]. The ACUITY risk score identified patients at increased risk for non-CABG-related bleeding and subsequent 1-year mortality.

Strategies to reduce the risk of bleeding and manage bleeding when it occurs are shown in Tables 2.11 and 2.12, respectively.

TABLE 2.11

Strategies to reduce the risk of bleeding

- Careful patient history, physical examination and assignment to therapy
- Appropriate dosing of antithrombotic drugs (consider age, renal function, weight)
- Short exposure to potent antithrombotic agents
- Use of fondaparinux is not indicated for PCI; alternative anticoagulants should be used during primary PCI
- Use of a PPI for gastric protection in patients at high risk
- For angiography/angioplasty:
  - consider radial artery access
  - minimize catheter size
  - remove sheaths as soon as possible
  - stop antithrombin immediately after the intervention
  - use bivalirudin
- Early response to bleeding, with careful alteration of medications depending on severity (note: early cessation of dual antiplatelet therapy is associated with a risk of stent thrombosis)
- Identification of retroperitoneal bleeding (perform CT scan in patients with back or leg pain, hypotension or progressive anemia)

PCI, percutaneous coronary intervention; PPI, proton pump inhibitor.

TABLE 2.12

Management of bleeding

Local hemostasis when possible

Minor bleeding

- Continue antithrombotic therapy if possible

Major bleeding

- Discontinue antithrombotic therapy
- Maintain volume status
- Avoid transfusion if possible (transfuse only when Hb < 80 g/L or Hct < 25%)
- Consider platelet transfusion; protamine for UH/enoxaparin
- Give prothrombin complex concentrate if high INR on warfarin
- Factor VII only if bleeding is severe or life-threatening

GP, glycoprotein; Hb, hemoglobin; Hct, hematocrit; INR, international normalized ratio; UH, unfractionated heparin.

Key points – diagnosis, risk stratification and decision-making

- Clinical recognition of acute coronary syndromes (ACS) requires a careful assessment of the clinical presentation and history, application of appropriate imaging techniques and measurement of biomarkers.
- A patient's symptom description is a critical diagnostic step, and typical symptoms such as chest heaviness, oppression and retrosternal burning are important angina symptoms.
- A 12-lead ECG should be performed and reviewed by an experienced clinician in all patients with suspected ACS within 10 minutes of first medical contact (i.e. on first contact with emergency medical services either outside or in hospital). If the likelihood of ACS is high but the 12-lead ECG is normal, a 17-lead ECG may be performed to reveal 'true posterior' ST-segment elevation myocardial infarction (STEMI).
- Early risk stratification is strongly recommended. Optimal risk stratification requires a multivariable approach. Clinical validated risk-stratification models such as the TIMI or GRACE risk scores are useful for assisting in management strategies and timing of invasive treatment in patients with suspected ACS.
- Invasive and non-invasive management strategies for ACS reduce the recurrence of ischemic events, but are associated with an increased risk of bleeding.
- Major bleeding and the need for transfusion are associated with an increased risk of in-hospital mortality as well as a long-term risk of death or MI; gastrointestinal and femoral access site bleeding are the most frequent bleeding complications.

Key references

Anderson JL, Adams CD, Antman EM et al. 2012 ACCF/AHA Focused Update Incorporated into the ACCF/AHA 2007 Guidelines for the Management of Patients With Unstable Angina/Non-ST-Elevation Myocardial Infarction. *J Am Coll Cardiol* 2013;61:e179–347.

Antman EM, Cohen M, Berninck PJ et al. The TIMI risk score for unstable angina/non-ST elevation MI: a method for prognostication and therapeutic decision making. *JAMA* 2000;284:835–42.

Braunwald E. Unstable angina and non-ST elevation myocardial infarction. *Am J Respir Crit Care Med* 2012;185:924–32.

CRUSADE bleeding score calculator. www.crusadebleedingscore.org, last accessed 04 November 2013.

Fitchett DH, Theroux P, Brophy JM et al. Assessment and management of acute coronary syndromes (ACS): a Canadian perspective on current guideline-recommended treatment– part 1: non-ST-segment elevation ACS. *Can J Cardiol* 2011;27 (Suppl A):S387–401.

Freynhofer MK, Tajsić M, Wojta J, Huber K. Biomarkers in acute coronary artery disease. *Wien Med Wochenschr* 2012;162:489–98.

Hamm CW, Bassand JP, Agewall S et al. ESC Guidelines for the management of acute coronary syndromes in patients presenting without persistent ST-segment elevation. *Eur Heart J* 2011;32:2999–3054.

Jneid H, Anderson JL, Wright RS et al. 2012 ACCF/AHA Focused Update of the Guideline for the Management of Patients With Unstable Angina/Non–ST Elevation Myocardial Infarction (Updating the 2007 Guideline and Replacing the 2011 Focused Update). *J Am Coll Cardiol* 2012;60:645–81.

O'Gara PT, Kushner FG, Ascheim DD et al. 2013 ACCF/AHA Guideline for the Management of ST-Elevation Myocardial Infarction. *J Am Coll Cardiol* 2013;61:e78–140.

Scirica BM. Acute coronary syndrome: emerging tools for diagnosis and risk assessment. *J Am Coll Cardiol* 2010;55:1403–15.

Steg PG, James SK, Atar D et al. ESC guidelines for the management of acute myocardial infarction in patients presenting with ST-segment elevation. *Eur Heart J* 2012;33:2569–619.

Thygesen K, Alpert JS, Jaffe AS et al. Writing Group on behalf of the Joint ESC/ACCF/AHA/WHF Task Force for the Universal Definition of Myocardial Infarction. Third universal definition of myocardial infarction. *J Am Coll Cardiol* 2012;60:1581–98.

The preferred approach to revascularization – percutaneous coronary intervention (PCI) or coronary artery bypass grafting (CABG) – depends on the extent and severity of the lesions as identified by coronary angiography, potential infarct complications, the patient's condition and comorbidities.

Percutaneous coronary intervention

The majority of PCIs are performed with the implantation of a stent(s) (Figure 3.1).

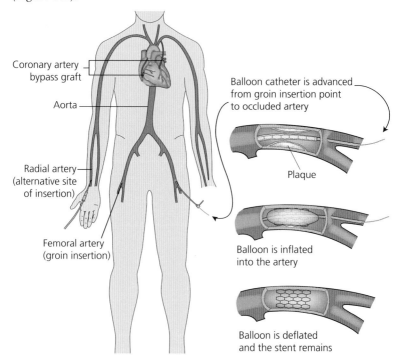

Figure 3.1 Percutaneous coronary intervention: a non-surgical method of opening narrowed coronary arteries using a balloon catheter to dilate the artery from within. A stent is usually implanted at the same time to maintain lumen integrity.

The procedure. During PCI, access into the femoral artery in the leg (or the radial artery or brachial artery in the arm) is created by a device called an 'introducer needle'. Once access is gained, a sheath is placed in the opening to keep the artery open and control bleeding. A long, flexible, soft plastic tube called a guiding catheter is advanced through the sheath over a guidewire. The tip of the guiding catheter is placed at the origin of the coronary artery. The guiding catheter also allows for iodine-based radiopaque dyes to be injected into the coronary artery, so that lesion location and severity can be precisely assessed using real-time radiographic visualization. This enables the cardiologist to estimate the size of the coronary artery and select the type of balloon catheter and coronary guidewire to use. A heparin or direct thrombin inhibitor is given to prevent clotting and maintain blood flow. A coronary guidewire, which is an extremely thin wire with a radiopaque flexible tip, is then inserted through the guiding catheter and into the coronary artery. Still using real-time radiographic visualization, the wire is guided through the coronary artery to the site of the stenosis or blockage. The tip of the wire is then passed across the blockage. The cardiologist controls the movement and direction of the guidewire by gently twisting the end that sits outside the patient.

While the guidewire is in place it acts as the pathway to and across the stenosis. An angioplasty balloon catheter, which is composed of a hollow tube, is inserted over the guidewire and is gently advanced forward until the deflated balloon is positioned across the blockage. The balloon is then inflated though a separate channel that sits coaxially along the catheter and the stenotic plaque is stretched and fractured, thus improving the luminal diameter and reducing the degree of stenosis. Usually, after balloon dilatation a stent is inserted to eliminate the problem of elastic recoil of the treated lesion.

Type of stent. Numerous factors affect the decision to use a bare-metal or a drug-eluting stent, including coronary anatomic features, clinical characteristics (e.g. diabetes), likely patient adherence to long-term dual antiplatelet therapy (DAPT), risk of bleeding with prolonged DAPT and the potential need for future surgical or other procedures that would require discontinuation of DAPT.

Several randomized clinical trials, which included patients with STEMI, have shown that drug-eluting stents reduce the risk of re-intervention compared with bare-metal stents, without having a significant impact on the risk of stent thrombosis, recurrent MI or death.

PCI is associated with superior restoration of myocardial blood flow, lower rates of reinfarction and mortality and less intracranial bleeding than pharmacological intervention with fibrinolytic therapy.

Choice of approach. The femoral approach has been widely adopted for PCI in the past. However, the radial approach has been increasingly favored in recent years because of potentially important advantages, including lower risk of major vascular complications and major bleeding, reduced length of stay after the procedure, reduced use of resources, and possibly lower mortality in high-risk patients such as those with STEMI. Moreover, the radial artery is superficial, which enables hemostasis to be achieved more readily. Bleeding at the site of radial access, radial artery injury and occlusion, increased radiation exposure, and the significant learning curve that is required to master the procedure before implementation of the radial approach as the standard method to achieve access in STEMI, are important considerations that need to be addressed when using the radial approach.

Coronary artery bypass grafting

Approximately 10% of patients with acute coronary syndromes (STEMI and NSTEMI) undergo CABG during initial hospitalization (Figure 3.2).

The procedure. CABG involves connecting, or grafting, a healthy artery (usually a mammary artery from the chest wall) directly to the coronary artery beyond the narrowing or blockage, or a vein to the coronary artery beyond the narrowing or blockage, and then connecting the vein to the aorta. Another potential artery used as a conduit is the radial artery. The bypass creates a new path for oxygen-rich blood to flow to the heart muscle. Single, double, triple, quadruple and quintuple (rare) bypasses can be made to a number of coronary arteries.

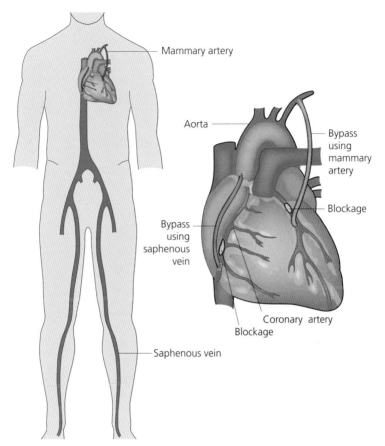

Figure 3.2 Coronary artery bypass grafting. Arteries or veins from elsewhere in the body are grafted to a coronary artery to bypass the narrowing or blockage.

For isolated CABG, the patient's heart is usually stopped and surgery is performed using cardiopulmonary bypass, aortic cross clamping and cardioplegic cardiac arrest (on-pump CABG). CABG can also be performed on a beating heart using various stabilization devices to provide a motionless surgical field (off-pump CABG). In general, off-pump CABG is not performed very frequently, unless there is heavy aortic calcification with a high risk of stroke associated with clamping. While avoidance of full-dose heparinization, potential hyperfibrinolysis and embolization of debris may reduce the incidence of CABG-related bleeding, particularly when performed during DAPT, stroke and postoperative respiratory complications, off-pump CABG may not be amenable to all stenotic lesions and may lead to repeat revascularizations or PCIs.

Approximately 15% of saphenous venous grafts occlude in the first year, and vein graft patency rates fall to approximately 75% and 60% 6 and 10 years after surgery, respectively. In contrast, 10-year patency for the internal thoracic artery is 85%.

Key points – coronary revascularization

- The preferred approach to revascularization depends on the extent and severity of the lesions, potential infarct complications and the patient's condition and comorbidities.
- Percutaneous coronary intervention (PCI) is associated with superior restoration of myocardial blood flow, lower rates of reinfarction and mortality and less intracranial bleeding than pharmacological intervention with fibrinolytic therapy.
- The use of drug-eluting stents is preferred as they reduce the risk of reintervention compared with bare-metal stents.
- Approximately 10% of patients with acute coronary syndromes undergo coronary artery bypass grafting during initial hospitalization.

Key references

Anderson JL, Adams CD, Antman EM et al. 2012 ACCF/AHA Focused Update Incorporated into the ACCF/AHA 2007 Guidelines for the Management of Patients With Unstable Angina/Non-ST-Elevation Myocardial Infarction: A Report of the American College of Cardiology Foundation/American Heart Association Task Force on Practice Guidelines. *J Am Coll Cardiol* 2013;61:e179–347.

Houlind K. On-pump versus off-pump coronary artery bypass surgery: what is the status after ROOBY, DOORS, CORONARY and GOPCABE? *Future Cardiol* 2013;9:569–79.

Levine GN, Bates ER, Blankenship JC et al. 2011 ACCF/AHA/SCAI Guideline for Percutaneous Coronary Intervention: a report of the American College of Cardiology Foundation/American Heart Association Task Force on Practice Guidelines and the Society for Cardiovascular Angiography and Interventions. *Circulation* 2011;124:e574–651.

Rao SV, Bernat I, Bertrand OF. Remaining challenges and opportunities for improvement in percutaneous transradial coronary procedures. *Eur Heart J* 2012;33:2521–6.

Wijns W, Kolh P, Danchin N et al.; Task Force on Myocardial Revascularization of the European Society of Cardiology (ESC) and the European Association for Cardio-Thoracic Surgery (EACTS); European Association for Percutaneous Cardiovascular Interventions (EAPCI). Guidelines on myocardial revascularization. *Eur Heart J* 2010;31:2501–55.

Surveys and registries suggest that the current incidence of unstable angina (UA) and non-ST-segment elevation myocardial infarction (NSTEMI), collectively known as non-ST-segment elevation acute coronary syndromes (NSTE-ACS), is higher than ST-segment elevation myocardial infarction (STEMI; see Chapter 5). Although the in-hospital mortality is higher in STEMI than UA/NSTEMI (7% vs 5%), the 6-month mortality rates are similar (12% vs 13%) and the 4-year mortality rates are two times higher in patients with UA/NSTEMI. In STEMI, most events occur before or shortly after presentation, but in UA/NSTEMI ischemic events continue over a longer period of time, possibly because patients with UA/NSTEMI tend to be older and have more comorbidities (Table 4.1).

TABLE 4.1

High-risk features for recurrent ischemic events after non-ST elevation acute coronary syndromes

Clinical	Electrocardiogram	Biomarker
• Multiple episodes of pain or documented ischemia	• Transient ST-segment elevation	• Troponin > 99th percentile reference level
• Hypotension, renal dysfunction, diabetes	• T-wave inversion > 2 mm in multiple precordial leads	
• Refractory ischemia with ECG changes despite treatment	• New left bundle branch block	
• Associated heart failure, prior revascularization	• Sustained ventricular tachycardia	

Adapted from Fitchett DH et al. 2011.

Clinical presentation

UA is defined by typical ECG changes (ST-segment depression, transient ST-segment elevation, T-wave inversion or some combination of these features) with ischemic symptoms (chest discomfort or anginal equivalent), while NSTEMI is defined by positive biomarkers of necrosis (e.g. troponin) without ST elevation (see Chapter 2) (Figure 4.1). NSTEMI can occur in the absence of ST-segment depression or T-wave inversion, and in some cases the ECG may show only non-specific changes or may even be normal.

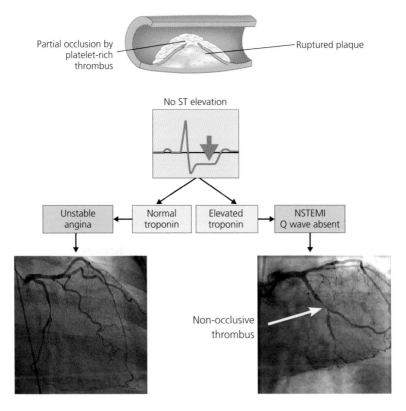

Figure 4.1 Characteristics of non-ST elevation acute coronary syndromes, as defined by ECG findings, the presence or absence of biomarkers and the degree of coronary occlusion (as seen on coronary angiography). NSTEMI, non-ST-segment elevation myocardial infarction; UA, unstable angina.

There are three principal clinical presentations of UA/NSTEMI:

- rest angina – occurs when the patient is at rest and usually lasts for more than 20 minutes
- new-onset severe angina – present for less than 2 months
- increasing angina – recent (secondary) destabilization of previously stable angina, increasing in intensity, duration and/or frequency.

Causes

The causes of UA/NSTEMI are shown in Table 4.2. Some patients can have two or more causes. The most common cause is a platelet-rich thrombus at the site of vascular injury, most often due to plaque rupture or endothelial erosion (see Chapter 1).

TABLE 4.2

Causes of unstable angina/non-ST-segment elevation myocardial infarction

- Thrombus or thromboembolism
  - occlusive thrombus, usually with collateral vessels
  - partial thrombus on pre-existing plaque
  - distal microvascular thromboembolism from plaque-associated thrombus
  - thromboembolism from plaque erosion
  - non-plaque-associated coronary thromboembolism
- Dynamic obstruction of epicardial and/or microvascular vessels (coronary spasm)
- Progressive mechanical obstruction to coronary flow
- Coronary arterial inflammation
- Coronary artery dissection (rare)

General management principles

UA/NSTEMI treatment strategies must equally address the acute phase as well as long-term management by:

- relieving angina and improving myocardial perfusion
- preventing thrombosis propagation
- stabilizing the vulnerable plaque
- attenuating the risk of developing long-term recurrent ischemic events (see Table 2.1).

Patients with UA/NSTEMI who are hemodynamically stable should be admitted to an inpatient unit for bed rest, continuous rhythm monitoring and careful observation for recurrent ischemia. Patients with continuing discomfort and/or hemodynamic instability should be hospitalized in a coronary care unit capable of providing continuous rhythm monitoring, frequent assessment of vital signs and mental status, and rapid defibrillation for ventricular fibrillation.

Conservative versus invasive treatment. One of the key early decisions in the treatment of UA/NSTEMI is whether to perform a cardiac catheterization (invasive management) and if so, when to proceed. Patients with hemodynamic compromise or symptoms refractory to medical therapy require immediate cardiac catheterization, except in those with serious comorbidities or contraindications (e.g. liver or pulmonary failure, cancer) to an invasive procedure. Otherwise, the decision is based upon an assessment of risk (see Chapter 2). Patients with high risk should be considered for early invasive management, while a conservative strategy is indicated for low-risk patients (Table 4.3).

An overview of the conservative and invasive treatment strategies for patients with UA/NSTEMI is provided in Figure 4.2.

Assessment of left ventricular function. Regardless of the strategy, an assessment of left ventricular (LV) function is recommended because treatment with angiotensin-converting enzyme (ACE) inhibitors and beta-blockers improves outcomes in patients with impaired LV function. When heart failure or diabetes mellitus is present, aldosterone antagonists are indicated.

57

TABLE 4.3

Patient characteristics to guide invasive or conservative treatment strategies

Invasive
- Recurrent angina/ischemia at rest with low-level activities despite intensive medical therapy
- Elevated cardiac troponins
- New/presumably new ST-segment depression
- Signs/symptoms of heart failure or new/worsening mitral regurgitation
- Hemodynamic instability
- Sustained ventricular tachycardia
- Percutaneous coronary intervention within past 6 months
- Previous coronary artery bypass graft surgery
- High risk score (e.g. TIMI, GRACE)
- Reduced left ventricular function (LVEF < 40%)

Conservative
- Low risk score (e.g. TIMI, GRACE)
- Patient/physician preference in the absence of high-risk features

GRACE, Global Registry of Acute Coronary Events; LVEF, left ventricular ejection fraction; TIMI, Thrombolysis in Myocardial Infarction.

Once the coronary angiogram has been obtained, a left ventriculogram will provide an estimate of LV function. When coronary angiography is not scheduled/performed, echocardiography, nuclear ventriculography, or MRI or CT angiography can be used to evaluate LV function. Echocardiography is most commonly performed since it reveals similar important clinical information, including ejection fraction, mitral insufficiency, ventricular septum defect, aortic stenosis and pericardial effusion.

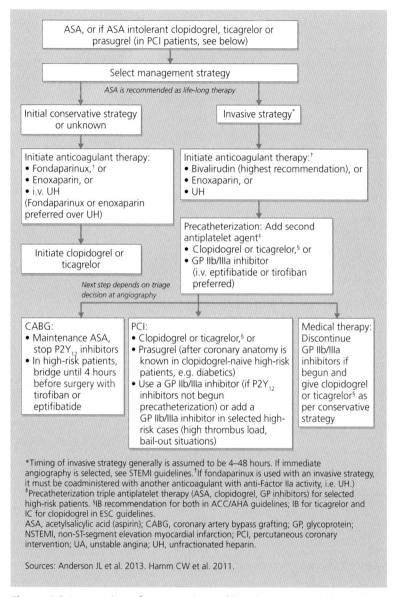

Figure 4.2 An overview of conservative and invasive treatment strategies for patients with likely or definite UA/NSTEMI. Note that the ACC/AHA and ESC guidelines provide different levels of evidence for the use of antithrombotic agents in NSTEMI patients. For information on these differences and the reasons, see Huber K and Lip GY 2013.

Invasive treatment

Increasingly, physicians are initiating an early invasive strategy in patients without contraindications, with coronary angiography within 24 hours of admission followed promptly by revascularization (see Chapter 3). The rationale for this more aggressive approach is the protective effect of revascularization on ischemic outcomes in high-risk patients. The decision to initiate a conservative strategy is guided by the absence of high-risk features, with angiography reserved for patients with recurrent ischemia or a high-risk stress test despite medical therapy.

In the absence of a randomized study comparing an early versus delayed strategy for coronary artery bypass grafting (CABG), the general consensus is to wait for 48–72 hours in patients who have had a culprit lesion PCI and have additional severe coronary artery disease (CAD). In patients needing CABG, scheduling should also be based on coronary anatomy. For example, patients with critical left main artery stenosis, ongoing ischemia symptoms, ventricular arrythmias and hemodynamic instability should receive timely operations.

Bleeding risk. Although pre-treatment with a triple or dual antiplatelet regimen may cause increased bleeding in the individual patient, a recent meta-analysis suggests that surgery-related bleeding decreases in these patients as surgical experience increases. In patients who require emergency surgery before the washout period of antiplatelet agents is completed, platelet transfusions, antifibrinolytics, off-pump CABG and use of recombinant factor VII (in extreme cases) may be employed to curtail bleeding.

Antithrombotic therapy

Since platelet function and coagulation play pivotal roles in the generation of a clot at the site of plaque rupture (see Chapter 1) and in subsequent ischemic events, a combination of antiplatelet and anticoagulant agents (together known as antithrombotic therapy) is the cornerstone of treatment for patients with ACS (Figure 4.3). However, the choice, initiation and duration of treatment depend on the severity of CAD, comorbid diseases, the clinical setting of

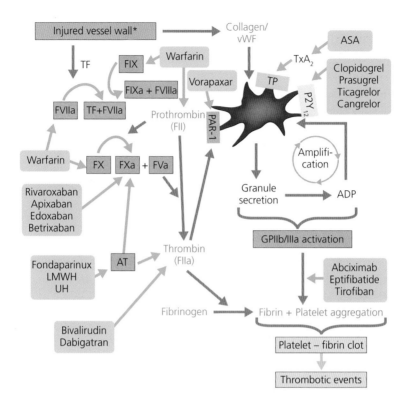

Figure 4.3 Modes of action of antithrombotic therapy. Antiplatelet therapy: acetylsalicylic acid (ASA; aspirin) inhibits thromboxane (Tx) A_2 generation and subsequently TxA_2-induced platelet aggregation. $P2Y_{12}$ receptor inhibitors (clopidogrel, prasugrel, ticagrelor, cangrelor) inhibit ADP-induced platelet aggregation (ADP is a major agonist). Abciximab, eptifibatide and tirofiban block the binding of fibrinogen to the glycoprotein (GP)IIb/IIIa receptor and prevent the final common pathway of platelet aggregation. Anticoagulant therapy: rivaroxaban, apixaban and other direct oral anticoagulants directly inhibit factor (F)Xa. Fondaparinux, low-molecular-weight heparin (LMWH) and unfractionated heparin (UH) bind to antithrombin (AT) and enhance the inhibition of thrombin or FXa to varying degrees. Bivalirudin and dabigatran directly inhibit thrombin. Warfarin inhibits the synthesis of vitamin K-dependent coagulation factors. *Denuded endothelium or plaque rupture due to percutaneous coronary intervention or acute coronary syndrome. ADP, adenosine diphosphate; PAR-1, platelet protease-activated receptor for thrombin; $P2Y_{12}$, platelet receptor for ADP; TF, tissue factor; TP, platelet receptor for thromboxane; TxA_2, thromboxane A_2; vWF, von Willebrand factor.

61

intervention (elective, acute or urgent intervention) and the type of stenting (bare-metal or drug-eluting). Proper risk assessment is essential to determine an optimal antithrombotic strategy that achieves a maximal antithrombotic effect associated with an acceptable bleeding risk (see Chapter 2).

Antiplatelet therapy

Currently approved antiplatelet strategies for ACS include acetylsalicylic acid (ASA; aspirin), $P2Y_{12}$ receptor inhibitors and GPIIb/IIIa inhibitors. Simultaneous inhibition of cyclo-oxygenase (COX)-1 and $P2Y_{12}$ by ASA and clopidogrel, respectively, has been shown in both preclinical and large-scale clinical studies to have a more potent antithrombotic effect than ASA alone. These pivotal findings form the basis for current therapeutic recommendations in ACS. However, with improved invasive technologies and concomitant treatments that address modifiable cardiovascular risk factors, ischemic event rates are falling in clinical trials and therefore the efficacy of treatment strategies that uniformly employ more potent platelet inhibition may also decrease in the future.

Acetylsalicylic acid (aspirin) is the bedrock of ACS antiplatelet treatment strategies and is indicated for both primary and secondary prevention.

Mechanism of action. The antithrombotic property of ASA is primarily attributed to irreversible acetylation of the platelet COX-1 enzyme. Subsequently, both the generation of thromboxane $(Tx)A_2$ and TxA_2-induced platelet aggregation are inhibited for the lifespan of the platelets. However, recent studies indicate that non-COX-1 effects of ASA in platelets and other pleiotropic effects may also contribute to the drug's antithrombotic properties. Platelet inhibition has been observed even before the appearance of ASA in the systemic circulation, suggesting that acetylation of platelet COX-1 takes place in the pre-hepatic circulation.

Dosing. The optimal dose for NSTE-ACS is controversial. In a meta-analysis, daily doses of 75–1500 mg showed similar clinical efficacy, while doses lower than 75 mg/day demonstrated a 50%

reduction in efficacy. In the CURRENT-OASIS-7 trial, which studied both the high and standard doses of clopidogrel and ASA in a 2 × 2 factorial design in patients with STEMI or NSTE-ACS, there were no significant differences in the 30-day outcomes of cardiovascular death, myocardial infarction (MI) or stroke, and no differences in major bleeding between ASA, 75–100 mg/day and 300–325 mg/day. A meta-analysis of secondary prevention studies also showed significant benefit associated with ASA treatment in the post-MI patient, including 21% reduction in serious vascular events (p<0.00001), 29% reduction in non-fatal MI (p=0.00003), 13% reduction in death related to coronary heart disease (p=0.04) and vascular death (p=0.03), 20% reduction in major coronary events (p=0.03) and no significant influence on any kind of stroke.

Current guidelines based on randomized trial protocols and clinical experience recommend immediate treatment with an initial dose of 162–325 mg (ACC/AHA) or 250(-500) mg (ESC), followed by indefinite 75–100 mg/day. When administered in conjunction with newer $P2Y_{12}$ receptor blockers, particularly ticagrelor, ASA, 75–100 mg/day is the preferred dosage; more than 100 mg of ASA may decrease the effectiveness of ticagrelor.

A non-enteric-coated tablet is recommended as initial therapy as it provides more rapid buccal absorption. Intravenous administration is also recommended in European countries. There is a strong rationale for concomitant use of ASA even if other antithrombotic drugs such as clopidogrel or warfarin are administered.

Side effects. The most common side effect of ASA treatment is gastrointestinal intolerance, which occurs in 5–40% of patients. Clopidogrel is recommended for patients who are allergic to, or who cannot tolerate, ASA. Withdrawal or discontinuation of ASA has been associated with recurrent ischemic events, including stent thrombosis. Concomitant administration of non-steroidal anti-inflammatory drugs (NSAIDs) should be avoided if possible, as NSAIDs, particularly ibuprofen, affect the access of ASA to its binding site within COX-1. Administration of ibuprofen should be delayed by at least 30 minutes after immediate-release ASA or at least 8 hours before ASA administration.

P2Y$_{12}$ receptor inhibitors inhibit adenosine diphosphate (ADP)-induced platelet activation and aggregation. At present, clinically used P2Y$_{12}$ receptor inhibitors include the thienopyridines (clopidogrel, prasugrel, ticlopidine) and the cyclopentyltriazolopyrimidine ticagrelor (Table 4.4). European guidelines, based on the TRITON-TIMI and PLATO trial results, recommend ticagrelor for all patients at moderate-to-high risk of ischemia (e.g. elevated troponin) and prasugrel for P2Y$_{12}$-receptor-naïve patients (especially diabetics) in whom coronary anatomy is known and who are proceeding to PCI, whereas clopidogrel is recommended only in patients who cannot receive prasugrel or ticagrelor.

Clopidogrel became the favored thienopyridine in the late 1990s because of the side effects associated with ticlopidine (rash, nausea, neutropenia, thrombocytopenia). It has demonstrated clinical efficacy in multiple large-scale trials and is now widely used in clinical practice. It is extensively used in dual antiplatelet therapy (DAPT) in addition to ASA in high-risk patients with CAD.

Pharmacodynamic studies in patients undergoing stenting indicate that clopidogrel is associated with variable and moderate levels of irreversible platelet inhibition, with a delayed onset of effect (about 8 hours with 300 mg loading dose, about 4 hours with 600 mg loading dose and 5 days with 75 mg daily maintenance dose to achieve a steady state of about 50% irreversible inhibition of platelet function). The wide variability in antiplatelet response results in a substantial number of stented patients (approximately 1 in 3) with high on-treatment platelet reactivity, which is strongly linked to recurrent ischemic events. Moreover, clopidogrel metabolism is influenced by single-nucleotide polymorphisms (SNPs) of genes encoding cytochrome isoenzymes (*CYP2C19*2* in particular), concomitant administration of drugs that either compete or inhibit the same cytochrome isoenzymes associated with clopidogrel metabolism, and other factors such as smoking, increased bodyweight, renal dysfunction and diabetes.

A higher clopidogrel dose has been shown to reduce the prevalence of high platelet reactivity: a strategy of higher clopidogrel loading and maintenance doses in the CURRENT-OASIS-7 trial was associated

TABLE 4.4

Characteristics of the P2Y$_{12}$ receptor antagonists

	Clopidogrel	Prasugrel	Ticagrelor	Cangrelor
Structure	Thienopyridine	Thienopyridine	CPTP derivative	ATP analog
Metabolism	Prodrug	Prodrug	Direct*	Direct
Administration	Oral, od	Oral, od	Oral, bd	Intravenous
Conversion to active metabolite	15%	85%	90–100%*	–
Type of action	Irreversible	Irreversible	Reversibly binding	Reversible
Elimination half-life	*Active metabolite:* After 75 mg =0.3 hours	*Active metabolite:* After 10 mg=0.5 (0.3–2.3) hours After 60 mg loading dose =7.4 (2–14.6) hours	*Parent compound:* 7 hours *Active metabolite:* 9 hours	3–4 minutes
Time to steady inhibition[†]	4–8 hours/5 days	1 hour	2 hours	Immediate
Offset[‡]	5–7 days	Up to 9 days	5–7 days	Immediate
Level of inhibition at steady state	40–50% wide response variability	65–80%	65–80%	> 90%
Elimination	Urine 40% Feces 60%	Urine 68% Feces 27%	Urine ~30% Feces ~60%	Urine

*Active metabolite is equally effective. [†]Time to steady inhibition has been evaluated in healthy volunteers and patients with stable coronary artery disease; therefore, it may be prolonged in patients presenting with ACS as they may be hemodynamically compromised. [‡]Time for platelet function to recover. ATP, adenosine triphosphate; bd, twice daily; CPTP, cyclopentyltriazolopyrimidine; od, once daily.

with reduced stent thrombosis and combined clinical endpoint rates but an increased risk of major bleeding in high-risk patients. Clopidogrel therapy is pharmacodynamically effective in about 65% of patients; about one-third of patients will have high platelet reactivity that is influenced by the carriage of SNPs (see Chapter 7).

In addition to loss-of-function allele, clopidogrel has a diminished pharmacodynamic effect in patients treated with proton pump inhibitors (PPIs), particularly omeprazole. Although highlighted by regulators, the clinical importance of this pharmacodynamic interaction remains highly controversial. Therefore, routine use of a PPI is not recommended for patients with a lower risk of upper gastrointestinal bleeding, who have much less potential to benefit from prophylactic therapy.

Prasugrel is a third-generation thienopyridine associated with a rapid onset of action and superior active metabolite generation, resulting in less response variability, a lower prevalence of non-responsiveness, less drug-drug interaction, less influence of loss-of-function allele and greater inhibition of ADP-induced platelet aggregation than clopidogrel.

In the TRITON-TIMI-38 trial, prasugrel plus ASA was associated with a 19% reduction in the primary composite endpoint of cardiovascular death, non-fatal MI and non-fatal stroke at a median 14.5-month follow-up compared with clopidogrel plus ASA in patients with NSTE-ACS and STEMI undergoing planned PCI. The benefit of prasugrel was mainly driven by a reduction in MIs. However, there were significantly increased key safety endpoints of TIMI major bleeding, including life-threatening and fatal bleeding, in patients treated with prasugrel. Prasugrel demonstrated a sustained reduction in the primary endpoint compared with clopidogrel (9.3% vs 11.2%, relative risk reduction=18%; p=0.002) in patients with NSTE-ACS who were clopidogrel naive after the first diagnostic angiogram and whose coronary anatomy was known, and in patients with STEMI in whom the agent could be used before the diagnostic angiogram and in patients pre-treated with clopidogrel. Prasugrel was especially effective in patients with diabetes and high-risk patients with recurrent thromboembolic events, and in reducing stent thrombosis. Loss-of-function allele SNPs did not appear to influence clinical outcomes during prasugrel treatment in a genetic substudy of the TRITON trial.

A maintenance dose of up to 5 mg/day has been approved by the US Food and Drug Administration (FDA) in patients weighing less than 60 kg or those older than 75 years of age due to a potential increased risk of bleeding.

Prasugrel is not recommended in patients with active pathological bleeding or a history of transient ischemic attacks (TIAs) or stroke. Prasugrel should not be initiated in patients likely to undergo urgent CABG. When possible, prasugrel should be discontinued at least 7 days before any surgery. In the TRILOGY trial, in patients with UA/NSTEMI who did not undergo revascularization, prolonged treatment with prasugrel was not associated with a reduced rate of major cardiovascular events compared with clopidogrel. However, this study demonstrated that a maintenance dose of 5 mg in individuals weighing less than 60 kg was safe, with lower non-CABG-related TIMI major bleeding incidences than clopidogrel. The ACCOAST trial demonstrated that pretreatment with prasugrel, 30 mg, in NSTEMI patients scheduled for catheterization was not effective in reducing the rate of major ischemic events up to 30 days but increased the rate of major bleeding complications.

Ticagrelor is a cyclopentyltriazolopyrimidine associated with a rapid onset of action, a greater level of inhibition that persists during maintenance therapy and a more rapid offset of pharmacodynamic action compared with clopidogrel. Ticagrelor therapy is also associated with greater platelet inhibition than clopidogrel in both clopidogrel responders and non-responders. Ticagrelor is extremely effective in reducing high on-treatment platelet reactivity within 30 minutes of therapy. Moreover, pharmacodynamic effect and clinical efficacy are not influenced by *CYP2C19* genetic polymorphisms.

In the PLATO trial, ticagrelor was associated with a significant reduction in the primary efficacy endpoint at 30 days compared with clopidogrel (4.8% vs 5.4%; p=0.045) and its superiority was maintained for 12 months, with a 16% relative risk reduction. A 17% relative reduction in the primary endpoint was observed in the 43% of patients who had NSTEMI (11.4% vs 13.9%). One of the most remarkable observations of the PLATO trial was the significant reduction in all-cause mortality associated with ticagrelor therapy.

There were no differences between ticagrelor- and clopidogrel-treated patients in the primary safety endpoint of major bleeding, as defined by either the study protocol or TIMI criteria. However, this analysis included perioperative bleeding complications in patients referred for coronary bypass surgery (10% of the total cohort). Although patients in the ticagrelor group were allowed to undergo CABG within 24–72 hours of discontinuing the study medication (versus 5 days in the clopidogrel group), the rate of CABG-related bleeding events was similar between the two groups. The rate of non-CABG-related major bleeding events was higher after ticagrelor treatment (4.5% vs 3.8%; p=0.026 and 2.8% vs 2.2%; p=0.025, for protocol and TIMI study group defined bleeding events, respectively).

Despite superior outcomes for ticagrelor across the rest of the international PLATO trial, the drug did not demonstrate a superior clinical effect in the North American patient population. This was attributed to the influence of the relatively high dosage (325 mg/day) of ASA used in this population. In addition, ticagrelor did not demonstrate a superior effect in patients with UA.

Potential side effects include an increase in spontaneous major bleedings, dyspnea and bradycardia; dyspnea and bradycardia-related effects have been attributed to the effect of ticagrelor on the inhibition of adenosine reuptake.

Cangrelor, an adenosine triphosphate (ATP) analog, is a parenteral direct-acting reversible $P2Y_{12}$ inhibitor with very rapid onset and offset pharmacodynamics (within minutes). In the CHAMPION-PCI and CHAMPION-PLATFORM trials, in which patients undergoing PCI were randomly assigned to therapy with cangrelor or placebo, cangrelor was not superior to placebo in reducing the primary endpoint of death, MI or ischemia-driven revascularization at 48 hours. In the BRIDGE trial, cangrelor resulted in a higher rate of maintenance of platelet inhibition than placebo among patients who discontinued thienopyridine therapy before surgery. In the CHAMPION-PHOENIX trial, cangrelor therapy was associated with a significantly reduced rate of ischemic events, including stent thromboses, during PCI, with no significant increase in severe bleeding.

Elinogrel is a direct-acting reversible $P2Y_{12}$ receptor antagonist. It is a first-in-class sulfonylurea that was administered either intravenously or orally. The choice of both parenteral and oral administration was hoped to facilitate a smooth transition from immediate to long-term therapy. The development of elinogrel has been stopped recently because of unfavorable efficacy and adverse side effects.

Thrombin receptor antagonists. Inhibition of the interaction between thrombin and protease-activated receptor (PAR)-1 may further attenuate ischemic events in selected patients treated with DAPT. Two major PAR-1 blockers have been studied: vorapaxar and atopaxar. In preclinical studies, inhibition of thrombin-mediated platelet activation by a PAR-1 inhibitor, in general, has added to the antithrombotic efficacy of ASA and clopidogrel without increasing bleeding.

The development of atopaxar has been stopped recently due to lack of significant benefits. Also, the TRACER study (vorapaxar versus placebo in addition to DAPT in NSTEMI-ACS) was stopped due to major bleeding, including intracranial hemorrhage, in the patient group receiving triple therapy. In the TRA 2P TIMI-50 secondary prevention trial, inhibition of PAR-1 with vorapaxar reduced the risk of cardiovascular death or ischemic events in patients with stable atherosclerosis who were receiving standard therapy. However, it increased the risk of moderate or severe bleeding, including intracranial hemorrhage. Accordingly, the future of vorapaxar is still under consideration but its use might be of interest for predefined patient groups.

Glycoprotein IIb/IIIa inhibitors. The pharmacological agents that directly and reversibly (plasma half-life of approximately 2 hours) block the binding of fibrinogen to the glycoprotein (GP) IIb/IIIa receptor (the final common pathway of platelet aggregation) are more effective in inhibiting platelet aggregation than any oral antiplatelet strategy. In addition to inhibition of platelet aggregation, GPIIb/IIIa inhibitors induce platelet disaggregation and may attenuate microembolization and the release of vasoconstrictors. The three GPIIb/IIIa inhibitors approved for intravenous administration, abciximab, eptifibatide and tirofiban, have different pharmacodynamic properties (see below). All of the GPIIb/IIIa inhibitors have been associated with an increase in bleeding compared with treatment with heparin alone. According to recent international guidelines GPIIb/IIIa inhibitors should be administered to patients with ACS undergoing PCI and when there is evidence of high thrombus load and/or slow or no reflow, or high risk of thrombotic complications. Recommended dosing is shown in Table 4.5.

Abciximab is a recombinant monoclonal antibody that binds to the GPIIb/IIIa receptor with high affinity, and also to the vitronectin receptor present in platelets, smooth muscle cells, monocytes and leukocytes and to the macrophage (MAC)-1 receptor present in leukocytes. An important side effect of abciximab, as well as eptifibatide and tirofiban, is thrombocytopenia.

Tirofiban is a peptidomimetic derivative of tyrosine that selectively and reversibly blocks the GPIIb/IIIa receptor by mimicking the RGD sequence (arginine-glycine-aspartate). Compared with abciximab, tirofiban has less affinity for the GPIIb/IIIa receptor and a shorter biological half-life (90–120 minutes) that depends on renal clearance.

Eptifibatide is a cyclic heptapeptide with a modified KGD sequence (lysine-glycine-aspartate) that reversibly blocks the GPIIb/IIIa receptor. Eptifibatide specifically binds to the GPIIb/IIIa receptor with low affinity and dissociates rapidly from the receptor, causing platelet aggregation to return to baseline in about 8 hours.

Clinial trial results. Most of the clinical trials demonstrating a favorable net clinical efficacy for GPIIb/IIIa inhibitor therapy pre-dated the era of early invasive therapy, PCI with uniform or near uniform stenting, and thienopyridine pretreatment. These older studies supported the upstream use of a GPIIb/IIIa inhibitor in combination with ASA and an anticoagulant in high-risk patients with ACS.

The ACUITY trial examined the optimal strategy for the use of GPIIb/IIIa inhibitors in moderate- and high-risk NSTE-ACS patients undergoing early invasive therapy. Bivalirudin alone, compared with heparin and a GPIIb/IIIa inhibitor, demonstrated non-inferiority in

TABLE 4.5

Dosing schedules for intravenous glycoprotein IIb/IIIa inhibitor therapy

Drug	Initial medical treatment	During PCI		After PCI
		Patient received initial medical treatment	Patient did not receive initial medical treatment	
Abciximab	–		0.25 mg/kg i.v. bolus; MD: 0.125 µg/kg/min (10 µg/min maximum)	Continue MD infusion for 12 hours
Eptifibatide	180 µg/kg i.v. bolus; MD: 2.0 µg/kg/min; reduce infusion by 50% in patients with estimated creatinine clearance < 50 mL/min	Continue infusion	180 µg/kg i.v. bolus, followed 10 mins later by second 180 µg/kg i.v. bolus; MD: 2.0 µg/kg/min; reduce infusion by 50% in patients with estimated creatinine clearance < 50 mL/min	Continue MD infusion for 18–24 hours (up to 72 hours maximum)
Tirofiban	LD: 0.4 µg/kg/min for 30 mins MD: 0.1 µg/kg/min; reduce rate of infusion by 50% in patients with estimated creatinine clearance < 30 mL/min	Continue infusion	LD: 0.4 µg/kg/min for 30 mins MD: 0.1 µg/kg/min; reduce rate of infusion by 50% in patients with estimated creatinine clearance < 30 mL/min	Continue MD infusion for 18–24 hours (up to 72 hours maximum)

LD, loading dose; MD, maintenance dose.

terms of the rate of the composite ischemia endpoint, significantly reduced rates of major bleeding and was associated with greater net clinical benefit. The ACUITY trial also demonstrated significantly lower major bleeding in the deferred-use group (at the time of angiography/PCI) versus the upstream group (at presentation and before angiography). In a subanalysis of patients who were not pretreated with a thienopyridine before PCI, the use of a GPIIb/IIIa inhibitor was associated with fewer ischemic events than bivalirudin therapy.

In the EARLY ACS trial, high-risk NSTE-ACS patients were randomized to receive either early routine administration of eptifibatide (double bolus followed by standard infusion) or delayed provisional eptifibatide at the time of PCI in addition to ASA and clopidogrel. There was no difference in the primary endpoint at 96 hours (9.3% vs 10%, OR: 0.92; p=0.23) and a non-significant decrease in the secondary endpoint (all-cause death or MI within 30 days) in patients in the early therapy arm versus patients in the delayed GPIIb/IIIa inhibitor arm. However, early routine eptifibatide administration was associated with a greater risk of TIMI major or minor bleeding, increased severe or moderate bleeding on the GUSTO bleeding scale and increased rates of red blood cell transfusion. The lack of significant efficacy and increased bleeding in the trial have affected recent guidelines for routine early GPIIb/IIIa inhibitor administration in NSTE-ACS patients.

The choice of upstream or deferred administration remains controversial, because true early administration (i.e. at the time of emergency department presentation) has never been achieved in a clinical trial despite the goal of testing the utility of 'early' administration. Various studies have indicated that GPIIb/IIIa inhibitors should only be used concomitantly with ASA and/or heparin in acute settings of ACS. The increasing use of the new antiplatelet agents prasugrel or ticagrelor in NSTE-ACS may further reduce the need for GPIIb/IIIa receptor blockers but this has not yet been addressed in specific randomized controlled trials. Novel strategies such as intracoronary administration, bolus-only strategy or short infusion of GPIIb/IIIa inhibitors are being studied, and evidence so far has suggested a benefit in reducing bleeding complications.

Anticoagulants

Anticoagulants can be classified as parenteral or oral (based on their administration route) or direct or indirect inhibitors (based on their target of action). Warfarin is not recommended routinely in all patients with ACS, but chronic oral anticoagulation with warfarin is recommended to attenuate thromboembolism or stroke in ACS patients with deep vein thrombosis, pulmonary embolism and atrial fibrillation.

Direct oral anticoagulants (DOACs) have been developed for long-term therapy mainly as an alternative to warfarin in patients with atrial fibrillation.

Major anticoagulants used in the treatment of NSTE-ACS are:
- indirect thrombin inhibitors that enhance the effects of antithrombin – unfractionated heparin (UH) and low-molecular-weight heparins (LMWHs)
- indirect Xa inhibitors that enhance the effects of antithrombin – LMWHs and fondaparinux
- direct thrombin inhibitors – dabigatran and bivalirudin
- direct factor Xa-inhibitors (xabans) – apixaban, rivaroxaban, edoxaban, betrixaban, otamixaban.

Indirect thrombin and Xa inhibitors

Unfractionated heparin is a heterogeneous mixture of polysaccharide molecules. The pentasaccharide sequence of UH binds to antithrombin and enhances the inhibition of thrombin and also factor Xa. UH binds plasma protein strongly, leading to unpredictable levels of free heparin in the circulation. UH therefore exhibits a significant variability in antithrombotic effects and requires close monitoring. In several randomized trials, UH has been associated with lower rates of death or MI than ASA alone. Most of the benefits of UH are short term and may be due to a rebound effect observed after discontinuation. Its other disadvantages include the need for continuous intravenous administration and the infrequent but serious complication of immunogenic heparin-induced thrombocytopenia. Due to the limitations of UH, LMWHs were developed with the goal of providing improved anticoagulation.

Low-molecular-weight heparins have less direct effect on thrombin and more effect on factor Xa, and less plasma binding, better bioavailability, less platelet activation and a lower risk of immune-mediated thrombocytopenia than UH. LMWH therapy can be administered subcutaneously on a weight basis and does not require dose adjustments or monitoring. The benefit of LMWH therapy may be more pronounced in the setting of a conservative strategy as demonstrated in older trials, whereas there was no observed benefit with LMWH in a recent trial (enoxaparin) in the setting of an early invasive strategy. Overall, in patients with ACS, LMWHs are superior to UH in decreasing the risk of major adverse cardiac events, despite a mild increase in bleeding. Patients with renal insufficiency may require lower-dose LMWHs since they are renally cleared. LMWHs are divergent agents and cannot be compared on a 1:1 basis. To date, the best investigated LMWH in cardiology is enoxaparin.

Fondaparinux, a factor Xa inhibitor, is a synthetic pentasaccharide that binds (reversibly with high affinity) to antithrombin III, thereby catalyzing the antithrombin III-mediated inhibition of factor Xa. Fondaparinux is administered subcutaneously and is rapidly absorbed, is completely bioavailable and has a predictable dose-dependent response. It can be administered in a fixed dose subcutaneously (2.5 mg once daily) and weight-based adjustment or routine monitoring is not necessary. It does not significantly interact with any cells or other plasma proteins and therefore does not affect platelet function or cause thrombocytopenia.

Fondaparinux is an effective primary antithrombotic agent in a conservative strategy for ACS and in thrombolysis in acute MI. It is not an optimal alternative to heparin or bivalirudin in NSTE-ACS within an invasive strategy (during angiography and PCI an additional bolus of UH, 85 IU/kg, is recommended).

Direct thrombin inhibitors act by binding to thrombin (both fluid-phase and fibrin-bound) and blocking the thrombin-induced conversion of fibrinogen to fibrin and the activation of FV, FVII, FIX and platelets. The latter functions are responsible for the amplification of thrombin generation. Direct thrombin inhibitors inhibit the activity of fibrin-bound thrombin. They have limited interaction with plasma proteins, making dosing and bioavailability much more predictable. These pharmacological properties make the direct thrombin inhibitors attractive alternatives to heparin as primary antithrombotic therapy in ACS patients.

The major direct thrombin inhibitors available are dabigatran, agratroban and bivalirudin.

Bivalirudin has demonstrated comparable anti-ischemic efficacy to and fewer bleeding complications than UH plus a GPIIb/IIIa inhibitor in several trials (REPLACE-2, ACUITY and HORIZONS). International guidelines recommend bivalirudin as a first-line anticoagulant in patients with ACS undergoing coronary intervention.

Dabigatran is an oral compound without liver toxicity (as was the case for ximelagatran). Dabigatran therapy was associated with significant benefits compared with warfarin in patients with non-valvular atrial fibrillation. It has been tested in a phase II dose-finding and safety trial (RE-DEEM) without substantial benefit in ACS patients and will therefore most likely not be further developed for this indication.

Direct factor Xa inhibitors apixaban, rivaroxaban, darexaban and otamixaban have been, or, are currently being, investigated in patients with ACS, either in the acute phase during intervention (otamixaban, TAO study) or in secondary prevention after the acute event (apixaban, APPRAISE trials; rivaroxaban, ATLAS trials; darexaban, RUBY-I trial).

Apixaban is an oral, selective, reversible and direct factor Xa inhibitor. It is absorbed rapidly, reaching maximal plasma concentrations after 3 hours, and the drug is cleared with a terminal plasma half-life of 8–14 hours. Since it is metabolized by hepatic CYP3A4, concomitant treatment with potent inhibitors of CYP3A4 is contraindicated. In the ARISTOTLE trial, apixaban was superior to warfarin in preventing stroke or systemic embolism, caused less bleeding and resulted in lower mortality in patients with non-valvular atrial fibrillation. In the APPRAISE-2 trial, the addition of apixaban, 5 mg twice daily, to standard DAPT (ASA and clopidogrel) in high-risk ACS patients was associated with increased major bleeding events but no significant reduction in recurrent ischemic events.

Rivaroxaban is an oral, direct factor Xa inhibitor with high oral bioavailability, rapid onset of action and a half-life of 7–10 hours. Rivaroxaban has been successfully tested in patients with non-valvular atrial fibrillation (ROCKET-AF trial) compared with warfarin. In the ATLAS ACS-TIMI 46 trial, the addition of rivaroxaban to ASA or DAPT in patients stabilized after an ACS increased bleeding in a dose-dependent manner and reduced major ischemic outcomes. In the ATLAS ACS-2 trial, the addition of rivaroxaban to DAPT, at doses lower than used for atrial fibrilliation, was associated with a significant reduction in the composite endpoint of death from cardiovascular causes, MI or stroke (26% reduction; p=0.008) but there was an increased risk of major bleeding (2.1% vs 0.6%; p<0.001) and intracranial hemorrhage (0.6% vs 0.2%; p=0.009) but not the risk of fatal bleeding in patients with a recent ACS. Rivaroxiban has been approved for use in Europe and is under review by the FDA for use in ACS.

Anticoagulant regimens. If a primarily conservative strategy is planned (e.g. in low-risk patients), fondaparinux, 2.5 mg subcutaneously once daily, or enoxaparin, 1 mg/kg subcutaneously twice daily, are the treatments of choice. UH, 60 IU/kg intravenous bolus, followed by an infusion (controlled by activated partial thromboplastin time), is also possible and frequently used in a 'real-world' setting.

In patients with an intermediate-to-high risk (e.g. troponin-positive, recurrent angina, dynamic ST changes, diabetes, renal dysfunction, early post-MI angina, previous PCI < 6 months, prior CABG, intermediate or high GRACE score), an early invasive strategy is preferable to a primarily conservative approach and should be performed within 24 (–48) hours. In general, the initial anticoagulant should be continued (except after initial therapy with fondaparinux; see below).

If treatment was started with enoxaparin and the intervention is performed less than 8 hours after the last subcutaneous application, no additional bolus is necessary; if enoxaparin was initiated 8–12 hours before the planned intervention (1 mg/kg subcutaneously; 0.75 mg/kg in patients older than 75 years), a 0.3 mg/kg intravenous bolus should be added; a 0.5 mg/kg intravenous bolus should be given if the last subcutaneous application of enoxaparin was more than 12 hours before the intervention.

Infusion should be continued during the procedure if UH (bolus plus infusion) was started before catheterization. Repeated activated clotting time measurements may be useful; the target range should be 200–250 seconds with GPIIb/IIIa inhibitors and 250–350 seconds when GPIIb/IIIa inhibitors are not used.

In NSTE-ACS patients treated with bivalirudin, a 0.1 mg/kg intravenous bolus followed by an infusion of 0.25 mg/kg/hour should be given for the diagnostic angiogram. An additional intravenous bolus of 0.5 mg/kg and an increase of the consecutive infusion to 1.75 mg/kg/hour before PCI is recommended. Recent recommendations ask for a prolongation of infusion until 4 hours after the intervention.

If fondaparinux was administered before catheterization, UH, 85 IU/kg, should be given as soon as angiography and PCI is performed, because patients receiving fondaparinux alone are at increased risk of catheter-related thrombus formation.

Patients with a very high risk of atherothrombotic events (e.g. clinical or ECG signs of persistent ischemia, hemodynamic instability, refractory arrhythmias) should be immediately transferred to the cath lab. Further therapeutic options consist of monotherapy with bivalirudin (dosage as above) or UH, 60 IU/kg intravenous bolus, followed by infusion until PCI or enoxaparin, 0.5 mg/kg intravenously, respectively.

UH and enoxaparin should be stopped immediately after PCI, except in specific situations (e.g. thrombotic complication, atrial fibrillation), while infusion with bivalirudin may be maintained for up to 4 hours after the intervention in order to improve its early efficacy.

Non-antithrombotic therapy

An overview of the non-antithrombotic agents administered to patients with NSTE-ACS is given in Table 4.6. Bed chair/rest is recommended, with continuous ECG monitoring. Supplemental oxygen should be administered in patients with arterial saturation less than 90%, respiratory distress or features suggestive of a high hypoxemia risk. Pulse oximetry is useful for continuous measurement of oxygen saturation.

TABLE 4.6

Non-antithrombotic therapy

- Bed/chair rest with ECG monitoring
- Supplemental oxygen
- Sublingual nitroglycerin
- Intravenous nitroglycerin
- Beta-blockers
- Calcium-channel blockers
- ACE inhibitors
- ARBs

ACE, angiotensin-converting enzyme; ARB, angiotensin receptor blocker.

Nitrates. After denitration, nitroglycerin releases nitric oxide and relaxes smooth muscle cells in arteries, arterioles and veins. Peripheral venodilation ensues and is accompanied by a reduction in preload and a decrease in myocardial wall tension. Afterload reduction is more modestly reduced. The reduction in preload and afterload contributes to reduced myocardial oxygen demand. Nitroglycerin also dilates major epicardial coronary arteries and enhances flow in collateral vessels. Despite limited evidence of benefit on clinical outcome, nitroglycerin is widely used in patients with UA/NSTEMI. Patients often obtain relief from sublingual (0.4 mg every 5 minutes for 3 doses), oral or topical nitroglycerin administration, before assessing the need for intravenous nitroglycerin over the first 48 hours. In patients with refractory angina or heart failure, intravenous administration is preferred.

Nitroglycerin is contraindicated in patients who have received phosphodiesterase-5 inhibitors (sildenafil, vardenafil, tadalafil) within 24 hours, because of enhanced vasodilation and the potential resulting hypotension. Nitroglycerin is also contraindicated in patients with systemic hypotension, marked tachycardia and severe aortic valve stenosis.

Sydnonimines and potassium-channel activators are alternatives to nitroglycerin but have not yet been well studied in patients with ACS.

Beta-blockers. By blocking the beta-adrenergic receptor for catecholamines on the myocardial cell membrane, beta-blockers reduce sinus node rate, atrioventricular node conduction velocity, contractility and arterial blood pressure, reducing myocardial oxygen demand and cardiac work. Myocardial and collateral flows improve due to prolongation of diastolic time. Beta-blockers exert beneficial effects in all forms of CAD.

Evidence for the beneficial effects of beta-blockers in UA is based on limited randomized trial data, along with pathophysiological considerations and extrapolation from experience in stable angina and STEMI. Beta-blockers are recommended in NSTEMI patients, unless they have significantly impaired atrioventricular conduction and a history of asthma or acute left ventricular dysfunction. In general, the recommendation is to start with oral therapy. Early intravenous beta-blocker therapy should be avoided in hemodynamically unstable patients and patients with heart failure but should be considered at the time of admission for hemodynamically stable patients with hypertension or tachycardia.

Calcium-channel blockers. By attenuating calcium transport into cells, calcium-channel blockers inhibit contraction of the myocardium (thereby reducing myocardial oxygen demand) and inhibit smooth muscle cell contraction, resulting in vasodilation and improvement in myocardial blood flow. There are three subclasses of calcium-channel blockers that cause varying degrees of vasodilation, a decrease in myocardial contractility and a delay in atrioventricular conduction:

- dihydropyridines (nifedipine, amlodipine)
- benzothiazepines (diltiazem)
- phenylalkylamines (verapamil).

There is no evidence of a mortality benefit, so calcium-channel blockers are not routinely administered as first-line therapy in patients with UA/NSTEMI, but rather used as third-line anti-ischemic agents after nitrates and beta-blockers or in patients for whom the use of beta-blockers are contraindicated.

Inhibitors of the renin-angiotensin-aldosterone system. The mortality benefits observed with the administration of angiotensin-converting enzyme (ACE) inhibitors favor the use of these drugs in all patients with UA/NSTEMI. ACE inhibitors should be administered within 24 hours to patients with congestive heart failure or an ejection fraction less than 40%. Long-term use of ACE inhibitors is also indicated in patients with high-risk chronic CAD. Angiotensin receptor blockers (ARBs) are generally reserved for patients who are intolerant to ACE inhibitors. Valsartan and captopril are equally effective for patients at high risk of cardiovascular events after MI.

Ivabradine, which selectively inhibits the primary pacemaker current in the sinus node, and nicorandil, which has nitrate-like properties, are new drugs that are indicated in patients with NSTEMI.

High-risk patient groups

The elderly. Although the morbidity risk increases in a linear fashion with each decade after the age of 50, patients over 65 years or over 75 years are the two most common 'elderly' groups defined. The prevalence of ACS-related complications such as heart failure, bleeding, stroke, renal failure and infections markedly increases with age. Common symptoms and signs observed in the elderly are shortness of breath (49%), diaphoresis (26%), nausea and vomiting (24%) and heart failure (41%), and the ECG in elderly patients with MI is more likely to be without ST elevation or ST depression (43%). Hypotension, bradycardia, renal failure and the risk of bleeding with antiplatelet agents and anticoagulants due to excessive dosing tend to be more common among elderly patients.

Elderly patients with NSTE-ACS are less likely to undergo an invasive strategy. However, reports from individual trials suggest that patients over 65 years of age derive substantial benefit from an invasive strategy but with an increase in the risk of major bleeding and the need for transfusions. Management strategies in elderly patients should be based on ischemic and bleeding risk, estimated life expectancy, comorbidities, quality of life, patient wishes, and the estimated risks and benefits of revascularization.

Women presenting with NSTE-ACS are generally older than their male counterparts and have a higher frequency of diabetes, hypertension, heart failure and other comorbidities. Atypical presentation, including dyspnea or symptoms of heart failure, is more common in women. Since registry data indicate that gender is not an independent risk factor for adverse cardiovascular events, it is recommended that women be evaluated and treated in a similar manner to men, with special attention being given to comorbid risk factors. Women tend to have higher rates of bleeding and non-obstructive CAD (with minimal atherothrombotic processes). GPIIb/IIIa inhibitors are primarily restricted to patients with elevated troponin levels and a high likelihood of CAD. A routine early invasive strategy is recommended primarily in high-risk women exhibiting ongoing ischemia and troponin elevation.

Patients with diabetes mellitus. Nearly one quarter of patients with UA/NSTEMI have diabetes. CAD is more severe among patients with diabetes and accounts for 75% of all deaths in this group. Moreover, diabetic patients have more extensive comorbidities such as hypertension, heart failure, LV hypertrophy, obesity and renal failure compared with non-diabetic patients. Diabetes is also an independent risk factor for recurrent ischemic events (death, MI or readmission for UA at 1 year: RR=4.9) in UA/NSTEMI patients.

The following are recommended in diabetic patients with UA/NSTEMI:
- aggressive glycemic control
- intravenous GPIIb/IIIa administration as part of initial medical management, which should be continued through the completion of PCI
- early invasive strategy in patients with single-vessel disease
- CABG for patients with multivessel disease and inducible ischemia.

Patients with chronic kidney disease. Renal dysfunction is a major risk factor for the development and progression of cardiovascular disease. The risk of cardiovascular and all-cause mortality increases exponentially with the progressive decrease of the glomerular filtration rate (GFR); a GFR lower than 60 mL/min/1.73m^2 is associated with a sudden increase in cardiovascular adverse events and these patients should undergo invasive evaluation and revascularization whenever possible. Renal dysfunction is also independently associated with bleeding risk in patients with ACS. Creatinine clearance and/or GFR should be estimated, and doses of renally cleared drugs adjusted, in patients with chronic renal failure.

Key points – unstable angina/non-ST-segment elevation myocardial infarction

- Although the in-hospital mortality is higher in patients with STEMI than those with UA/NSTEMI, the 6-month mortality rates are similar and the 4-year mortality rates are two times higher in patients with UA/NSTEMI.
- Early invasive strategy followed promptly by revascularization is increasingly preferred over conservative strategy.
- Antithrombotic therapy is a fundamental strategy in patients with UA/NSTEMI; however, proper risk assessment is essential to determine an optimal strategy that achieves a maximum anti-ischemic effect associated with an acceptable bleeding risk.
- Dual antiplatelet therapy with acetylsalicylic acid (ASA; aspirin) and a $P2Y_{12}$ receptor blocker is the standard of care in patients with UA/NSTEMI; however, optimal duration of therapy is controversial.
- Guidelines uniformly recommend starting all UA/NSTEMI patients (without contraindications) on an anticoagulant as soon as possible after presentation.
- The benefits of triple therapy of ASA, $P2Y_{12}$ receptor blocker and warfarin/oral anticoagulant have not been clearly established. The role of direct oral anticoagulants for long-term therapy is being studied in large-scale trials.
- Since patients with UA/NSTEMI have a high risk of recurrent ischemic events, active long-term management strategies are crucial.

Key references

Anderson JL, Adams CD, Antman EM et al. 2012 ACCF/AHA Focused Update Incorporated into the ACCF/AHA 2007 Guidelines for the Management of Patients With Unstable Angina/Non-ST-Elevation Myocardial Infarction: A Report of the American College of Cardiology Foundation/American Heart Association Task Force on Practice Guidelines. *J Am Coll Cardiol* 2013;61:e179–347.

Angiolillo DJ, Firstenberg MS, Price MJ et al.; BRIDGE Investigators. Bridging antiplatelet therapy with cangrelor in patients undergoing cardiac surgery: a randomized controlled trial. *JAMA* 2012;307:265–74.

Baigent C, Blackwell L, Collins R et al.; Antithrombotic Trialists' (ATT) Collaboration. Aspirin in the primary and secondary prevention of vascular disease: collaborative meta-analysis of individual participant data from randomised trials. *Lancet* 2009;373:1849–60.

Braunwald E. Unstable angina and non-ST elevation myocardial infarction. *Am J Respir Crit Care Med* 2012;185:924–32.

Fitchett DH, Theroux P, Brophy JM et al. Assessment and management of acute coronary syndromes (ACS): a Canadian perspective on current guideline-recommended treatment – part 1: non-ST-segment elevation ACS. *Can J Cardiol* 2011;27 (Suppl A):S387–401.

Giugliano RP, White JA, Bode C et al.; EARLY ACS Investigators. Early versus delayed, provisional eptifibatide in acute coronary syndromes. *N Engl J Med* 2009;360:2176–90.

Gurbel PA, Tantry US. Combination antithrombotic therapies. *Circulation* 2010; 121:569–83.

Hamm CW, Bassand J-P, Agewall S et al. ESC Guidelines for the management of acute coronary syndromes in patients presenting without persistent ST-segment elevation: The Task Force for the management of acute coronary syndromes (ACS) in patients presenting without persistent ST-segment elevation of the European Society of Cardiology (ESC). *Eur Heart J* 2011;32:2999–3054.

Huber K, Lip GY. Differences between ACC/AHA and ESC Guidelines on antiplatelet therapy in patients with acute coronary syndromes. *Thromb Haemost* 2013;110:11–13.

Jneid H, Anderson JL, Wright RS et al. 2012 ACCF/AHA Focused Update of the Guideline for the Management of Patients With Unstable Angina/Non–ST Elevation Myocardial Infarction (Updating the 2007 Guideline and Replacing the 2011 Focused Update). A Report of the American College of Cardiology Foundation/American Heart Association Task Force on Practice Guidelines. *J Am Coll Cardiol* 2012;60:645–81.

Lincoff AM, Bittl JA, Harrington RA et al.; REPLACE-2 Investigators. Bivalirudin and provisional glycoprotein IIb/IIIa blockade compared with heparin and planned glycoprotein IIb/IIIa blockade during percutaneous coronary intervention: REPLACE-2 randomized trial. *JAMA* 2003;289:853–63.

Mehta SR, Bassand JP, Chrolavicius S et al.; CURRENT-OASIS 7 Investigators. Dose comparisons of clopidogrel and aspirin in acute coronary syndromes. *N Engl J Med* 2010;363:930–42.

Mehta SR, Tanguay JF, Eikelboom JW et al.; CURRENT-OASIS 7 trial investigators. Double-dose versus standard-dose clopidogrel and high-dose versus low-dose aspirin in individuals undergoing percutaneous coronary intervention for acute coronary syndromes (CURRENT-OASIS 7): a randomised factorial trial. *Lancet* 2010;376:1233–43.

Roe MT, Armstrong PW, Fox KA et al.; TRILOGY ACS Investigators. Prasugrel versus clopidogrel for acute coronary syndromes without revascularization. *N Engl J Med* 2012;367:1297–309.

Scirica BM. Acute coronary syndrome: emerging tools for diagnosis and risk assessment. *J Am Coll Cardiol* 2010;55:1403–15.

Wallentin L, James S, Storey R et al. for the PLATO investigators. E ect of CYP2C19 and ABCB1 single nucleotide polymorphisms on outcomes of treatment with ticagrelor versus clopidogrel for acute coronary syndromes: a genetic substudy of the PLATO trial. *Lancet* 2010;376:1620–8.

ST-segment elevation myocardial infarction

Approximately 30% of all patients with acute coronary syndromes (ACS) have ST-segment elevation myocardial infarction (STEMI). Over the past decade, clinical outcomes for patients with STEMI have improved as a result of increased awareness, speed of diagnosis, and treatment with both reperfusion and adjuvant medical therapy. Despite these developments, thousands of STEMI patients fail to receive critical therapy in a timely fashion each year, and nearly 30% do not receive any reperfusion treatment.

Clinical presentation

STEMI is characterized by a typical rise of myocardial necrosis biomarkers and ST-segment elevation (or left bundle branch block; LBBB), ultimately progressing to Q-wave myocardial infarction (MI) (Figure 5.1). The diagnosis of STEMI is confirmed by evidence of myocardial necrosis based on ECG, biomarkers or pathological examination. Total occlusion of the culprit coronary artery is most often observed due to fibrin-rich thrombus formation. Concomitant vasoconstriction and microembolization play a more minor role in the pathophysiology. Fibrin-rich clot formation is important for the subsequent stabilization of the early and fragile platelet-rich thrombus that is more often observed alone in NSTEMI. Often, there may be a delay of up to 2 weeks between rupture of the plaque and its clinical manifestation as STEMI.

Myocardial necrosis following complete occlusion of the coronary artery develops 15–30 minutes after severe ischemia when there is no forward or collateral flow, and progresses as a 'wavefront' from the subendocardium to the subepicardium in a time-dependent fashion. At this time, reperfusion may save the myocardium from necrosis, and subnormal but persistent forward flow may extend the time window for myocardial salvage.

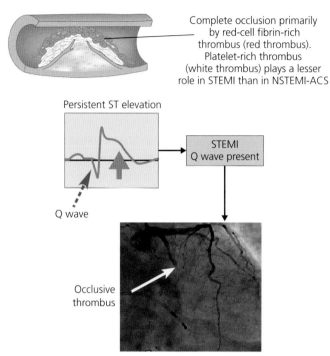

Figure 5.1 Characteristics of ST-segment elevation myocardial infarction (STEMI), as defined by the degree of coronary occlusion and characteristic ECG changes: pink arrow indicates elevation of ST segment; dotted blue arrow shows Q wave.

The amount of myocardial damage following infarction is dependent on:
- the area supplied (downstream) from the site of thrombotic vessel occlusion
- the duration and extent of occlusion
- the amount of blood supplied by collateral vessels to the affected tissue
- the demand for oxygen supply from the area at risk.

MIs can be clinically silent and unrecognized by the patient. These patients are more likely to be older, women, diabetic and/or have previous heart failure. Angiographic evidence of coronary thrombus formation (see Figure 1.2) may be seen in more than 90% of patients with STEMI but in only 1% of patients with stable angina and 35–75% of patients with unstable angina (UA) or non-ST-segment myocardial infarction (NSTEMI).

Usually, high levels of cardiac troponin can be observed for 7–10 days after STEMI. Following reperfusion, there may be an earlier rise in cardiac troponin levels, which reach a higher peak value due to rapid washout from the interstitium of the infarct zone, before rapid decline.

Causes

A higher frequency of STEMI in the early morning may be due to beta-adrenergic stimulation (increased vascular tone and blood pressure), hypercoagulability and platelet hyperreactivity. Vigorous physical exercise, emotional stress and medical or surgical illness also trigger plaque disruption and thrombosis. The thrombotic response to plaque disruption is dynamic: thrombosis and clot lysis, often associated with vasospasm, occur simultaneously, and may cause intermittent flow obstruction and distal embolization. The absence of complete healing of an aging plaque (incomplete re-endothelialization) and thrombus formation play important roles in the occurrence of sudden occlusive coronary thrombosis. In 25–30% of patients undergoing primary percutaneous coronary intervention (PCI), initial angiography shows a patent infarct-related artery. In these patients, it is presumed that spontaneous, endogenous lysis occurred before angiography.

Acute management

In the emergency department, the management of patients with suspected STEMI includes pain control, rapid identification of patients eligible for urgent reperfusion therapy, triaging lower-risk patients to the appropriate setting in the hospital and avoiding inappropriate discharge of patients with STEMI. Initial management includes acetylsalicylic acid (ASA; aspirin), sublingual nitroglycerin and intravenous beta-blockers, and morphine to control the pain. In patients with hypoxemia, oxygen should be administered by nasal prongs or face mask.

87

Reperfusion strategies

There are two reperfusion strategies available:
- mechanical (PCI)
- pharmacological (fibrinolytic).

Reperfusion should be performed as soon as possible in patients with ST elevation of at least 2 mm (0.2 mV) in two contiguous precordial leads or 1 mm in two adjacent limb leads or a presumed new LBBB. Patients without ST-segment elevation are not candidates for immediate pharmacological reperfusion but should receive anti-ischemic therapy and catheter-based therapy.

The goal for mechanical reperfusion is to achieve intracoronary balloon inflation within 90 minutes of the patient's arrival at hospital or first contact with the medical system (door [or FMC]-to-balloon time) (Figure 5.2). The goal of pharmacological reperfusion is to initiate fibrinolytic therapy within 30 minutes (door-to-needle time). It is recommended that early reperfusion (preferably primary PCI) should be performed within 12 hours of symptom onset in patients with the clinical presentation of STEMI (Figure 5.3) and for those with persistent ST-segment elevation or new or presumed new LBBB. There is no consensus as to whether PCI is beneficial in patients who present more than 12 hours after the onset of ischemia without clinical and/or ECG evidence of ongoing ischemia.

Early mortality risk assessment can be based on the TIMI (Thrombolysis in Myocardial Infarction) risk score for STEMI (see page 36). High-risk patients with cardiogenic shock or a very high TIMI risk (> 7) are likely to benefit from primary PCI more than fibrinolysis since there is evidence of a poorer lytic effect in the presence of hemodynamic compromise.

Percutaneous coronary interventions (see Chapter 3) during the early hours of STEMI can be divided into:
- primary PCI (first-line)
- facilitated PCI – PCI combined with pharmacological reperfusion therapy
- 'rescue PCI' after failed pharmacological reperfusion.

The patient should be immediately transferred to a hospital with PCI capabilities if there is any evidence of persistent occlusion, re-occlusion or reinfarction with recurrence of ST-segment elevation.

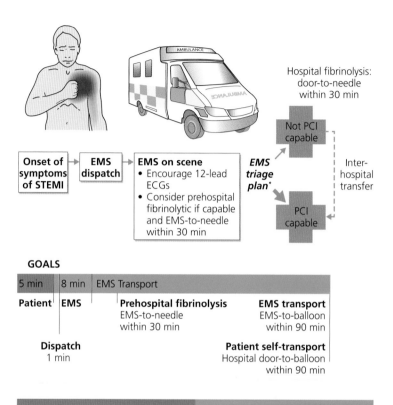

Figure 5.2 Options for transport of patients with ST-segment elevation myocardial infarction (STEMI) and initial reperfusion treatment. *It is preferable to transfer to a PCI-capable hospital if there are time-delay issues. EMS, emergency medical services; PCI, percutaneous coronary intervention.

Primary percutaneous coronary intervention is defined as angioplasty and/or stenting without prior or concomitant fibrinolytic therapy. It should be performed in hospitals with an established interventional cardiology program as a routine treatment option. This strategy is more effective in securing and maintaining coronary artery patency than fibrinolysis and avoids some of the bleeding risks of fibrinolysis (see above). Indications for primary PCI are shown in Table 5.1.

89

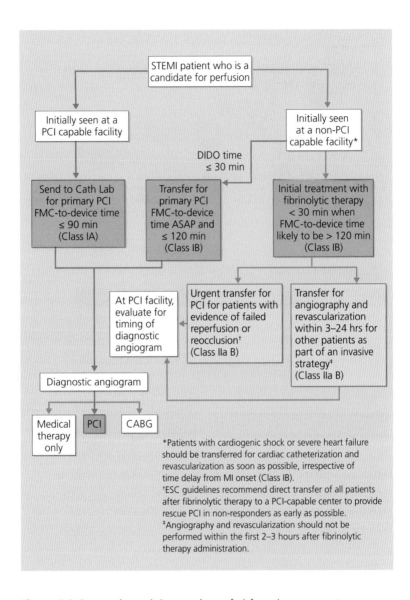

Figure 5.3 Care pathway (triage and transfer) for primary percutaneous coronary intervention (PCI) in patients with suspected ST-segment elevation myocardial infarction (STEMI). Red arrows and shaded boxes indicate preferred strategies. CABG, coronary artery bypass grafting; DIDO, door-in to door-out; FMC, first medical contact; MI, myocardial infarction.

Source: O'Gara PT et al. 2013;61:485–510.

TABLE 5.1

Indications for primary percutaneous coronary intervention in patients with STEMI

- Skilled cath lab available
  - First medical contact-to-balloon time or door-to-balloon time ≤ 90 mins (≤ 60 mins recommended in acute STEMI of < 2 hours' duration)
- High risk from STEMI (e.g. cardiogenic shock)
- Late presentation (> 12 hours after symptom onset) – primary PCI is preferred over fibrinolytic therapy
- More mature clot, less easily lysed by fibrinolytic drugs
- Contraindications for fibrinolytic therapy (high risk of bleeding and ICH)
- STEMI diagnosis in doubt

ICH, intracranial hemorrhage; PCI, percutaneous coronary intervention; STEMI, ST-segment elevation myocardial infarction.

Routine coronary stent implantation (see Chapter 3) in patients with STEMI decreases the need for target vessel revascularization and significantly reduces reinfarction rates compared with balloon angioplasty. Although previously it was suggested that rapid coronary artery thrombus aspiration in STEMI patients during catheterization may improve blood flow and restore ST-segment elevation, routine thrombus ASA (aspirin) before PCI, as compared with PCI alone, was not associated with reduced 30-day mortality among patients with STEMI in the recently published open-label TASTE trial.

Worse clinical outcomes have been observed in both randomized studies and registries when long delays have occurred before the primary PCI, i.e. increased time from symptom onset to first medical contact (FMC – ECG-confirmed diagnosis of STEMI), time from FMC to arrival in the cath laboratory, time from FMC to sheath insertion, and time from FMC to balloon inflation. The 'PCI-related time delay' is the theoretical difference between the time of FMC to balloon inflation minus the time from FMC to start of fibrinolytic therapy ('door-to-balloon' minus 'door-to-needle'; see Figure 5.2). The extent to which the PCI-related time delay (which may be between 60 and 120 minutes) diminishes the advantages of PCI over fibrinolysis has been the subject of many analyses and debates. Therefore, primary PCI (balloon inflation) should optimally be performed within 2 hours of FMC. In patients presenting early, with a large amount of myocardium at risk, the delay should be less than 60 minutes from FMC. Although much emphasis has been given to achieving lower FMC-to-balloon time in general practice, in-hospital and short-term mortality has remained virtually unaffected despite a significantly increased percentage of patients meeting the criteria of FMC-to-balloon time of 90 minutes or less (recently reported results from a registry of 95 007 STEMI patients).

Patients with contraindications to fibrinolytic therapy have a higher morbidity and mortality than those eligible for this therapy. Primary PCI is the preferred treatment for patients in shock. Except for patients in cardiogenic shock, only the culprit lesion should be dilated in the acute setting. Complete revascularization of the non-culprit lesions may be performed later depending on the remaining ischemia.

Facilitated (pharmaco-invasive) percutaneous coronary intervention. In order to bridge the PCI-related time delay, pharmacological reperfusion treatment can be delivered before a planned PCI during facilitated PCI. Full-dose lytic therapy, half-dose lytic therapy with a glycoprotein (GP)IIb/IIIa inhibitor, and full-dose GPIIb/IIIa inhibitor have all been studied, but there is no evidence of a significant clinical benefit with any of these strategies. During facilitated PCI, pre-PCI patency rates were higher without mortality benefit, but more bleeding complications were observed with lytic-based treatments. In some studies, the pre-PCI patency rates with upfront abciximab or high-bolus dose tirofiban (GPIIb/IIIa inhibitors) alone were higher than with placebo, but in general a reduction in hard clinical endpoints based on facilitation is still missing.

Rescue percutaneous coronary intervention is defined as PCI performed within 12 hours on a coronary artery that remains occluded despite fibrinolytic therapy. Non-invasive identification of failed fibrinolysis is challenging, but less than 50% ST-segment resolution in the lead(s) with the highest ST-segment elevations

60–90 minutes after the start of fibrinolytic therapy has increasingly been used as a surrogate marker.

Rescue PCI has been shown to be feasible and relatively safe. A recent meta-analysis showed that rescue PCI is associated with a significant reduction in heart failure and reinfarction and a trend towards lower all-cause mortality when compared with a conservative strategy, but with an increased risk of stroke and bleeding complications.

Rescue PCI should be considered when there is evidence of failed fibrinolysis based on clinical signs and insufficient ST-segment resolution (< 50%), if there is clinical or ECG evidence of a large infarct, and if the procedure can be performed within a reasonable time period (up to 12 hours after the onset of symptoms). An immediate transfer of patients to a PCI-capable center after initiation of fibrinolytic therapy usually helps to shorten the time until rescue PCI.

If rescue PCI is not available, there is a large infarct and the risk of bleeding is not high, a second administration of a non-immunogenic fibrinolytic agent (see above) may be considered, although readministration of a fibrinolytic agent has not been shown to be superior to conservative therapy.

STEMI networks. Geographic considerations and distribution of primary PCI centers mean that, for many regions in North America (and most countries in Europe), primary PCI can only be provided within the recommended time intervals for the majority of the population if systems are in place to optimize its application. In Europe, 20–95% of patients with STEMI undergo primary PCI, and numbers are increasing, a range that reflects local resources and capabilities. Unfortunately, of those who are referred for primary PCI, not all patients receive optimal mechanical reperfusion (i.e. FMC-to-balloon time of less than 90–120 minutes with the procedure performed in an experienced center with an experienced team). These findings argue for allocation of additional resources to establish and further expand STEMI treatment networks, as is being done in the 'Mission: Lifeline' program in the USA ('Stent for Life' activities in Europe). The key to success, however, begins with local organization of dedicated care providers in each community. With the agreement of all stakeholders and participants in optimized networks, financial, regulatory

93

and political barriers can be resolved, and prompt guidelines-recommended care becomes feasible, achievable and affordable.

Fibrinolytic therapy. An overview of the nine trials performed by the Fibrinolytic Therapy Trialists' Collaborative Group shows that approximately 30 early deaths are prevented per 1000 patients within 35 days for those treated with fibrinolytic therapy, and 20 deaths are prevented per 1000 patients when treatment is given 7–12 hours after symptom onset. These benefits were observed in patients with ST-segment elevation or LBBB at the time of presentation, irrespective of age, gender, blood pressure, heart rate or history of MI or diabetes. The available data support prehospital initiation of fibrinolytic treatment if reperfusion is indicated. Early fibrinolytic therapy is associated with similar outcomes to primary PCI, if early angiography and PCI were performed in those patients who needed intervention. The principal goal of fibrinolysis is prompt restoration of normal myocardial blood flow. Indications for fibrinolytic therapy are shown in Table 5.2.

Fibrinolytic agents are streptokinase, alteplase, reteplase and tenecteplase (Table 5.3); urokinase is also used infrequently in certain

---

TABLE 5.2

Indications for fibrinolytic therapy in patients with STEMI

- Early presentation (≤ 3 hours from symptom onset and delay to PCI)

- Primary PCI is not an option:
  - cath lab is occupied or unavailable within 90–120 minutes from first medical contact (when the diagnosis is made)

- Delay to primary PCI
  - FMC minus FMC-to-needle time > 1 hour
  - FMC-to-balloon time or door-to-balloon time > 90–120 minutes

FMC, first medical contact; PCI, primary coronary intervention; STEMI, ST-segment elevation myocardial infarction.

TABLE 5.3

Properties and dosing requirements of fibrinolytic agents

	Streptokinase	Alteplase	Reteplase	Tenecteplase
Mean plasma half-life (min)	Unavailable	3.5	14	17
Mean plasma clearance (min)	Unavailable	572	283	151
Dose	1.5 million units over 30–60 min i.v.	15 mg i.v. bolus 0.75 mg/kg over 30 min then 0.5 mg/kg over 60 min i.v. Total dosage not to exceed 100 mg	10 U + 10 U i.v. bolus given 30 min apart	Single i.v. bolus 30 mg if < 60 kg 35 mg if 60 to < 70 kg 40 mg if 70 to 80 kg 45 mg if 80 to < 90 kg 50 mg if > 90 kg
Fibrin specificity	None	++	+	++++
TIMI grade 3 flow at 90 min	32	54	60	63

i.v., intravenous; TIMI, thrombolysis in myocardial infarction (risk score).

areas of the world. These drugs enhance the conversion of plasminogen to plasmin, which subsequently lyses fibrin thrombi. Streptokinase is a non-fibrin-specific agent and is the least expensive, but it is least effective in achieving full reperfusion of the coronary artery (with TIMI grade 3 flow) and improving survival rates when compared with the fibrin-specific agents.

The newer fibrin-specific agents have longer half-lives and can be administered rapidly and as a bolus. The most widely used is tenecteplase, which is associated with less non-cerebral bleeding and less need for blood transfusion, but a similar 30-day mortality benefit to alteplase.

Adverse effects. Fibrinolytic therapy is associated with a small but significant increase in the risk of stroke, mainly confined to the first day after treatment. Early strokes are largely attributable to cerebral hemorrhage; later strokes are more frequently thrombotic or embolic. Advanced age, lower weight, female gender, previous cerebrovascular disease, and systolic and diastolic hypertension on admission are significant predictors of intracranial hemorrhage.

In the latest trials, intracranial bleeding occurred in 0.9–1.0% of the patients treated, whereas major non-cerebral bleeds (bleeding complications requiring blood transfusion or life-threatening) occurred in 4–13%. The most common sources of bleeding are procedure related. Independent predictors of non-cerebral bleeding are older age, lower weight and female gender.

Contraindications to fibrinolytic therapy are shown in Table 5.4.

Assessment of reperfusion is crucial to establish the successfulness of therapy. Flow in the culprit coronary artery is measured by a simple qualitative scale based on an angiographic measurement called the thrombolysis in myocardial infarction (TIMI) grading system.

- Grade 0 – complete occlusion of the infarct-related artery.
- Grade 1 – some penetration of the contrast material beyond the point of obstruction but without perfusion of the distal coronary bed.
- Grade 2 – perfusion of the entire infarct vessel into the distal bed but with flow that is delayed compared with that of a normal artery.

TABLE 5.4

Contraindications to fibrinolytic therapy

Absolute contraindications

- Hemorrhagic stroke or stroke of unknown origin at any time
- Ischemic stroke in preceding 6 months
- CNS trauma or neoplasms
- Recent major trauma/surgery/head injury (within preceding 3 weeks)
- Gastrointestinal bleeding within the last month
- Known bleeding disorder
- Aortic dissection
- Non-compressible punctures (e.g. liver biopsy, lumbar puncture)

Relative contraindications

- Transient ischemic attack in preceding 6 months
- Oral anticoagulant therapy
- Pregnancy or within 1 week postpartum
- Refractory hypertension (systolic blood pressure > 180 mmHg and/or diastolic blood pressure > 110 mmHg)
- Advanced liver disease
- Infective endocarditis
- Active peptic ulcer
- Prolonged or traumatic resuscitation

CNS, central nervous system.
Source: 2012 ESC STEMI Guidelines.

- Grade 3 – full perfusion of the infarct vessel with normal flow.

The main aim of the reperfusion strategy is to achieve TIMI grade 3, i.e. to ensure full perfusion of the infarct-related coronary artery. This gives far better results in terms of limiting infarct size, maintaining left ventricular (LV) function and reducing both short- and long-term mortality rates.

Additional assessment strategies include:

- TIMI frame count – angiographic assessment of the efficacy of fibrinolysis by counting the number of frames on the cine film required for dye to flow from the origin of the infarct-related artery to a landmark in the distal vascular bed.
- TIMI myocardial perfusion grade – determination of the rate of entry and exit of contrast dye from the microvasculature in the myocardial infarct zone.

Currently, angiographic assessment of epicardial flow is considered inadequate because of impaired microvascular perfusion, even when TIMI grade 3 flow and less than 50% coronary narrowing have been achieved. Evaluation of ST-segment resolution on ECG is a simple and readily available technique to assess reperfusion. A resolution of more than 50% of ST-segment elevation 60–90 minutes after the initiation of therapy is considered a good indicator of improved myocardial perfusion and is associated with enhanced recovery of LV function, reduced infarct size and improved prognosis. According to the ACC/AHA guidelines, it is reasonable to monitor the pattern of ST-segment elevation, cardiac rhythm and clinical symptoms during the 60–180 minutes after the initiation of fibrinolytic therapy (class IIa recommendation).

Non-invasive findings suggestive of successful reperfusion include relief of symptoms, maintenance or restoration of hemodynamic or electrical stability or both, and a reduction of at least 50% in the initial ST-segment elevation injury pattern as demonstrated by follow-up ECG 60–90 minutes after the initiation of therapy. In contrast, unrelenting ischemic chest pain, absence of resolution of the qualifying ST-segment elevation, and hemodynamic or electrical instability are generally indicators of failed pharmacological reperfusion and the need to consider rescue PCI.

Antithrombotic therapy

The major goals of antithrombotic therapy during STEMI are to establish and maintain patency of the infarct-related artery, limit the consequences of myocardial ischemia, enhance reperfusion, heal myocardial damage and attenuate recurrent adverse events. Further information on the drugs discussed below can be found in Chapter 4.

Antiplatelet therapy

Acetylsalicylic acid (aspirin) is recommended in all patients with STEMI as early as possible, with same initial dose as for UA/NSTEMI (see page 63), and low-dose ASA, 75–100 mg/day, continued indefinitely. In patients intolerant to ASA, clopidogrel is indicated as an alternative.

Clopidogrel. Recent European guidelines recommend the use of clopidogrel, a loading dose of 600 mg followed by a maintenance dose of 75 mg/day, only if prasugrel or ticagrelor are not available or contraindicated. Clopidogrel should be used as early as possible, in the ambulance or the emergency room depending on the local situation, for the biggest benefit.

Prasugrel. A loading dose of 60 mg followed by a maintenance dose of 10 mg, in combination with ASA, showed a statistical reduction of the combined primary endpoint and cardiovascular mortality when compared with clopidogrel in STEMI patients. Major bleeding complications were equal in the two study groups. In STEMI patients referred for primary PCI, international guidelines recommend that prasugrel should be administered as soon as possible. Although early use of a 60-mg loading dose (e.g. in the ambulance on the way to the catheter-equipped tertiary hospital) has not yet been investigated, this strategy has become standard practice in many STEMI networks.

Ticagrelor has also demonstrated greater efficacy than clopidogrel, with a similar severe bleeding rate (including perioperative bleedings), but it failed to demonstrate significant benefit over the comparator with respect to the combined clinical endpoint in a prespecified analysis of the STEMI subgroup.

Abciximab is the GPIIb/IIIa inhibitor most extensively studied in acute STEMI patients referred for primary PCI (used as a 0.25 mg/kg intravenous bolus followed by infusion of 0.125 µg/kg/min up to a maximum of 10 µg/min for 12 hours) in combination with unfractionated heparin (UH). The 'upstream' use of GPIIb/IIIa-blockers has no strong recommendation in current guidelines, because the only prospective randomized trial to investigate the pre- versus in-cath lab use of abciximab (FINESSE trial) was negative with respect to hard clinical endpoints. However, meta-analyses, registries and large post-hoc analyses have provided results in favor of an early use of abciximab, particularly in patients with fresh infarction (diagnosed and treated less than 3 hours after the onset of pain). Recently, it was shown that intracoronary administration of abciximab had no benefit over its intravenous application (AIDA-STEMI trial).

Dual antiplatelet therapy (DAPT). In the European guidelines, a combination of ASA and prasugrel or ticagrelor is recommended (over ASA and clopidogrel) in patients treated with PCI. DAPT is recommended for 9–12 months after ACS, independent of the type of stent used. However, the precise duration (6 months or more than 1 year) is still controversial and is being studied (Table 5.5). The results of the recently published PARIS registry indicate that in the real-world setting, optimal duration or cessation for DAPT is not uniform and also not yet clear. While most of the adverse events occurred while patients were taking DAPT, temporary DAPT interruption lasting up to 14 days was not associated with an increased rate of thrombotic events and also physician-guided cessation was associated with substantially fewer adverse events. At the same time, unanticipated antiplatelet therapy cessation may put patients at an increased risk for adverse events.

Gastric protection with a proton pump inhibitor should be considered for the duration of DAPT in patients at high risk of bleeding (Level IIaC evidence).

Anticoagulation. Bivalirudin monotherapy, 0.75 mg/kg as an intravenous bolus followed by infusion to 1.75 mg/kg/hour up to 4 hours, is recommended as a first-line anticoagulant in patients with ACS undergoing coronary intervention. In the HORIZONS-AMI trial, bivalirudin therapy alone was associated with significantly reduced 30-day and 3-year rates of major bleeding and a reduction in net adverse clinical events compared with heparin plus GPIIb/IIIa inhibitors in patients with STEMI undergoing primary PCI. Similar results were demonstrated in the recent EUROMAX trial, which studied pre-hospital use of bivalirudin versus heparin plus GP IIb/IIIa inhibitors. This trial further confirmed the preferred use of bivalirudin as an anticoagulant in STEMI patients undergoing primary PCI.

UH should be started with 60 IU/kg intravenous bolus when a GPIIb/IIIa inhibitor is used or with 100 IU/kg intravenous bolus

TABLE 5.5

Current guidelines for duration of antiplatelet therapy after ACS

2013 ACCF/AHA/SCAI guidelines

After bare-metal or drug-eluting stent implantation during primary PCI

Clopidogrel, 75 mg/day; or prasugrel, 10 mg/day (5 mg in elderly and/or underweight patients); or ticagrelor, 90 mg twice daily, for at least 12 months

After fibrinolytic therapy (conservative therapy)

ASA to be continued indefinitely, plus clopidogrel, 75 mg/day, for at least 14 days, up to 12 months

In patients undergoing PCI after fibrinolytic therapy

Clopidogrel, 75 mg/day; or prasugrel,*10 mg/day, for at least 12 months (after drug-eluting stent) or at least 30 days and up to 12 months (after bare-metal stent)

2012 ESC guidelines

DAPT (ASA and a P2Y$_{12}$ receptor antagonist)† in patients with STEMI undergoing primary PCI (for up to 12 months) or fibrinolysis (for up to 12 months) and in patients who have not undergone reperfusion therapy (for at least 1 month and up to 12 months). In addition, 1 month of DAPT in patients after bare-metal stenting and 6 months in patients after drug-eluting stenting

*Prasugrel should not be administered to patients with a history of prior stroke or transient ischemic attack. †Clopidogrel in patients after fibrinolytic therapy or no reperfusion therapy, or those with a contraindication against more effective P2Y$_{12}$ inhibitors. Prasugrel or ticagrelor in patients who have already received these drugs during primary PCI.
ASA, acetylsalicylic acid (aspirin); DAPT, dual antiplatelet therapy; PCI, percutaneous coronary intervention; STEMI, ST-segment elevation in myocardial infarction.
Adapted from O'Gara PT et al. 2013 (USA) and Steg PG et al. 2012 (Europe).

without GPIIb/IIIa inhibitors. UH should be stopped immediately after successful PCI unless specific indications make continued use necessary (e.g. left ventricular aneurysm and/or thrombus, atrial fibrillation, prolonged bed rest or deferred sheath removal). As long as patients need bed rest the use of prophylactic low-molecular-weight heparin (LMWH) to minimize the risk of venous thrombosis is recommended.

In the ATOLL trial, enoxaparin, 0.5 mg intravenous bolus, was compared with UH in STEMI patients undergoing primary PCI. In this superiority trial, enoxaparin failed to reach a statistical benefit with respect to the combined primary endpoint (cardiovascular death, re-MI, reintervention and severe bleeding after 30 days) but was superior to UH with respect to the different secondary endpoints. A possible explanation for not demonstrating superiority over UH was the fact that bleeding complications under enoxaparin were not statistically lower compared with UH, possibly due to radial access, which was used in more than 70% of the patients.

Fondaparinux is not recommended at all in primary PCI for acute STEMI patients because of concerns for catheter-related thrombus and interventional complications.

Anti-ischemic agents

Nitroglycerin is administered in STEMI patients to relieve ischemic pain and also as a vasodilator in patients with LV failure. Since the benefit of nitroglycerin administration has not been convincingly demonstrated, its routine use is not recommended.

In addition to nitroglycerin, morphine is an effective analgesic for the pain associated with STEMI. It has unpredictable absorption and is therefore routinely administered by repetitive (every 5 minutes) intravenous injection of small doses (2–4 mg) rather than by the subcutaneous administration of a larger quantity.

Beta-blockers. Intravenous beta-blockers are used in patients with STEMI regardless of the planned reperfusion strategy, but must be avoided in patients with hypotension or heart failure. Oral treatment should be considered during hospital stay and continued thereafter in all STEMI patients without contraindications, and is indicated in patients with heart failure or LV dysfunction. A commonly employed regimen is oral metoprolol, 50–100 mg twice daily or 200 mg daily (class I indication).

Other agents. Unlike beta-blockers, calcium antagonists are of little value in the acute management of STEMI. However, verapamil may be considered for secondary prevention in patients with absolute contraindications to beta-blockers and no heart failure.

Administration of angiotensin-converting enzyme (ACE) inhibitors should be considered in all patients without contraindications, and within the first 24 hours of STEMI in patients with impaired ejection fraction (EF ≤ 40%) or evidence of heart failure, diabetes or an anterior infarct. An angiotensin receptor blocker, preferably valsartan, is an alternative in patients who are intolerant to ACE inhibitors.

High-dose statins should be initiated or continued early after admission in all STEMI patients without contraindication or history of intolerance, regardless of initial cholesterol values. A fasting lipid profile should be obtained in all STEMI patients as soon as possible after presentation, and reassessment of LDL cholesterol considered after 4–6 weeks to ensure a target of 1.8 mmol/L (70 mg/dL) has been reached.

Aldosterone antagonists (e.g eplenerone) are indicated in patients with an ejection fraction less than 40% and heart failure or diabetes, provided they do not have renal failure or hyperkalemia.

Key points – ST-segment elevation myocardial infarction

- Immediate recognition of STEMI with timely initiation of reperfusion therapies is associated with improved outcomes.
- The selection of reperfusion strategy in STEMI (pharmacological versus invasive) is critically dependent on the time from onset of symptoms, mortality risk of STEMI and bleeding risk.
- Primary percutaneous coronary intervention (PCI) is the preferred choice of revascularization in STEMI patients if it can be offered within 90–120 minutes of diagnosis.
- Prasugrel and ticagrelor have superseded clopidogrel as the gold standard in dual antiplatelet therapy.
- In the European guidelines, bivalirudin is the anticoagulant of choice during primary PCI, while enoxaparin has its merits as an adjuvant to thrombolytic therapy. Whereas, in the US guidelines there is no general preference for bivalirudin over unfractionated heparin and there is no recommendation for enoxaparin.

Exercise-based rehabilitation is recommended. It should include aerobic exercise of moderate intensity (e.g. running, swimming, walking, cycling) for 30 minutes at least five times a week.

Key references

Agewall S, Cattaneo M, Collet JP et al.; ESC Working Group on Cardiovascular Pharmacology and Drug Therapy and ESC Working Group on Thrombosis. Expert position paper on the use of proton pump inhibitors in patients with cardiovascular disease and antithrombotic therapy. *Eur Heart J* 2013;34:1708–13.

Huber K, Goldstein P, Danchin N et al. Enhancing the efficacy of delivering reperfusion therapy: a European and North American experience with STEMI networks. *Am Heart J* 2013;165:123–32.

Levine GN, Bates ER, Blankenship JC et al. 2011 ACCF/AHA/SCAI Guideline for Percutaneous Coronary Intervention. A Report of the American College of Cardiology Foundation/American Heart Association Task Force of Practice Guidelines and the Society for Cardiovascular Angiography and Interventions. *J Am Coll Cardiol* 2011;58:e44–122.

O'Gara PT, Kushner FG, Ascheim DD et al. 2013 ACCF/AHA guideline for the management of ST-elevation myocardial infarction: a report of the American College of Cardiology Foundation/American Heart Association Task Force on Practice Guidelines. *Circulation* 2013;127:e362–425. Executive summary *J Am Coll Cardiol* 2013;61:185–510.

Reimer KA, Lowe JE, Rasmussen MM, Jennings RB. The wavefront phenomenon of ischemic cell death. 1. Myocardial infarct size vs duration of coronary occlusion in dogs. *Circulation* 1977;56:786–94.

Steg PG, James SK, Atar D et al. Task Force on the management of ST-segment elevation acute myocardial infarction of the European Society of Cardiology (ESC). ESC Guidelines for the management of acute myocardial infarction in patients presenting with ST-segment elevation. *Eur Heart J* 2012;33:2569–619.

Steg PG, van 't Hof A, Hamm CW et al.; the EUROMAX Investigators. Bivalirudin started during emergency transport for primary PCI. *N Engl J Med* 2013; Oct 30 [Epub ahead of print].

Wijns W, Kolh P, Danchin N et al. Guidelines on myocardial revascularization: The Task Force on Myocardial Revascularization of the European Society of Cardiology (ESC) and the European Association for Cardio-Thoracic Surgery (EACTS). *Eur Heart J* 2010; 31:2501–55.

Despite reduced mortality during the acute phase of acute coronary syndromes (ACS) because of improved and timely reperfusion strategies, patients with coronary artery disease (CAD), particularly patients with non-ST-segment elevation myocardial infarction (NSTEMI), remain at heightened risk for long-term recurrent cardiovascular events. The potential underlying mechanisms include advancing age, ischemic complications caused by residual or progressive atherosclerotic CAD, arrhythmias resulting from the trigger of latent ischemia or arising from the re-entrant substrate provided by the infarct scar, and heart failure.

The goal of secondary prevention strategies is to reduce cardiovascular death, recurrent myocardial infarction (MI), the burden of angina and other ischemic events. Numerous hospital-based (cardiac rehabilitation) and cost-effective home-based secondary prevention programs have been shown to improve processes of care, coronary risk factor profiles and quality of life. However, internationally, patient access to these programs is low (around 30%), particularly in those groups with the greatest need for risk factor reduction, i.e. those with diabetes, dyslipidemia, hypertension, obesity, smoking or a family history of CAD.

More than 90% of the risk of CAD is associated with modifiable risk factors, and detailed US and European guidelines are available for the long-term management of specific coronary risk factors and left ventricular dysfunction (see Key references). Nevertheless, patients with CAD do not achieve treatment targets regarding lifestyle changes, risk factor modification and therapeutic strategies, and there are huge gaps in applying current evidence to routine practice. Non-adherence to secondary prevention guidelines is a major problem. Measures to improve adherence to medications and healthy lifestyle choices, improved awareness and education programs targeting both patients and healthcare providers are needed.

Smoking cessation

Smokers are twice as likely to present with ST-segment elevation myocardial infarction (STEMI) as non-smokers. The goal must be to completely stop smoking as well as avoid exposure to environmental tobacco smoke. Once the patient's smoking status has been assessed, they should be referred to a smoking cessation program. The patient's family should also be encouraged to stop smoking to help with avoidance of secondhand smoking. The patient should be advised to quit and avoid passive smoking at all subsequent visits. Counseling, nicotine replacement, buproprion and antidepressants are all helpful elements in smoking rehabilitation efforts. For further information see *Fast Facts: Smoking Cessation.*

Blood pressure control

The goal should be to achieve a blood pressure of 140/90 mmHg, or less than 130/80 mmHg if the patient is diabetic or has chronic kidney disease. In addition to lifestyle modifications (reduced salt intake, increased physical activity, weight control and alcohol moderation), pharmacotherapy (beta-blockers, angiotensin-converting enzyme [ACE] inhibitors, or angiotensin receptor blockers [ARBs]) is recommended. For further information see *Fast Facts: Hypertension.*

Diet and weight control

The goal of weight management control is to achieve a body mass index (BMI) of 18.5–24.9 kg/m² and waist circumference less than 40 inches for men and less than 35 inches for women. BMI and/or waist circumference should be assessed at every visit, and the healthcare provider should consistently encourage weight maintenance or reduction through an appropriate balance of physical activity, caloric intake and formal behavioral programs. A reduction in bodyweight of 5–10% from baseline is an achievable initial goal. Healthcare providers are recommended to encourage patients to exercise regularly, regardless of age.

Non-hydrogenated unsaturated fat (the predominant form of dietary fat), whole grain (the predominant form of carbohydrate), fruits and vegetables and omega-3 fatty acids (from fish, fish oil supplements or plant sources) offer significant protection against

CAD. European recommendations for a 'heart healthy' diet are shown in Table 6.1.

For further information see *Fast Facts: Obesity.*

Lipid management

In general, the goal of lipid management is to achieve a target level of less than 100 mg/dL LDL cholesterol; for very high-risk patients (e.g. patients presenting with acute STEMI or CAD patients with diabetes) a further reduction of LDL cholesterol to less than 70 mg/dL should be considered. If triglyceride levels are 200 mg/dL or more, the goal for non-HDL cholesterol (total cholesterol–HDL cholesterol) should be less than 130 mg/dL; lower than 100 mg/dL for very high-risk patients is reasonable. Provided there are no contraindications, these targets can usually be reached by use of a highly effective high-dose statin such as atorvastatin, 80 mg, or rosuvastatin, 20 mg, initiated during the index hospital stay.

At least a 30–40% reduction in LDL cholesterol levels is recommended when LDL-lowering medications are used. Lowering

TABLE 6.1

Dietary guidelines for a healthy heart

- Eat a wide variety of foods
- Adjust calorie intake to avoid obesity
- Increased consumption of:
  - fruit and vegetables
  - wholegrain cereals and bread
  - fish (especially oily varieties)
  - lean meat
  - low-fat dairy products
- Replace saturated and trans fats with monounsaturated and polyunsaturated fats from vegetable and marine sources
- Reduce total fats (of which less than one-third should be saturated) to 30% of total calorie intake
- Reduce salt intake if blood pressure is raised.

LDL cholesterol is also beneficial in patients with renal complications. In the Study of Heart and Renal Protection (SHARP) daily doses of simvastatin, 20 mg, plus ezetimibe, 10 mg, safely reduced the incidence of major atherosclerotic events in a wide range of patients with advanced chronic kidney disease.

For further information see *Fast Facts: Hyperlipidemia.*

Physical activity

Exercise can reduce the anxiety associated with life-threatening illness and improve patients' self-confidence, cardiorespiratory fitness and exercise capacity. All patients should be risk assessed with a physical activity history and/or exercise test to guide prognosis and prescription. At least 30 minutes of moderate aerobic exercise (e.g. brisk walking) 7 days per week (minimum 5 days per week) is recommended. Medically supervised rehabilitation programs are useful for high-risk patients.

Physical activity improves four key mechanisms, which are considered to be important mediators of a reduced cardiac event rate:
- improves endothelial function
- reduces the progression of coronary lesions
- reduces thrombogenic risk
- increases the number of collateral vessels.

Diabetes management

The goal of diabetes management is to maintain a glycosylated hemoglobin (HbA_{1c}) concentration of less than 7%, and should be coordinated in conjunction with the patient's primary care provider and diabetes specialist. For further information see *Fast Facts: Diabetes Mellitus.*

Treatment of depression

Depression is a frequent consequence of STEMI and also one of the most important predictors for the development of ACS. It has been reported that approximately 15% of patients who have had a MI experience major depressive disorder, while a further 15–20% exhibit mild to moderate depression. Moreover, post-MI depression is more likely to be associated with poorer adherence to medication and utilization of health services, increased morbidity and suicide risk, poorer risk factor profiles for congestive heart disease, and reduced quality of life and survival.

Depression remains poorly recognized and managed in patients with ACS. Secondary prevention programs for depression are usually delivered face-to-face in clinic- or hospital-based settings; however, access to and participation in these programs is low. Psychological-based therapies and treatment with selective serotonin reuptake inhibitors have been shown to reduce depression in ACS patients, especially those with recurrent depression. Cognitive behavioral therapy (CBT) has been shown to be particularly favorable in improving depression outcomes for cardiac patients and is recommended in international guidelines. For more information see *Fast Facts: Depression.*

Key points – secondary prevention of coronary artery disease

- Patients with acute coronary syndromes, particularly NSTEMI, remain at heightened risk for long-term recurrent cardiovascular events.
- The goal of secondary prevention strategies is to reduce cardiovascular death, recurrent myocardial infarction, the burden of angina, and other ischemic events.
- More than 90% of the risk of coronary artery disease (CAD) is associated with modifiable risk factors. Secondary prevention trials are therefore mainly targeting the modifiable risk factors such as diabetes, dyslipidemia, hypertension, obesity and smoking.
- Despite many secondary prevention programs, patients with CAD do not achieve treatment targets regarding lifestyle changes, risk factor modification and therapeutic strategies, and there are huge gaps in applying evidence to routine practice.
- Strict adherence to medications, improved awareness and education programs targeting patient and healthcare providers are needed.

References

Haddad M, Gunn J. *Fast Facts: Depression*, 3rd edn. Oxford: Health Press, 2011.

Haslam D, Wittert G. *Fast Facts: Obesity*. Oxford: Health Press, 2009.

MacGregor GA, Kaplan NM. *Fast Facts: Hypertension*, 4th edn. Oxford: Health Press, 2010.

O'Neil A, Hawkes AL, Chan B et al. A randomised, feasibility rial of a tele-health intervention for acute coronary syndrome patients with depression ('MoodCare'): study protocol. *BMC Cardiovasc Disord* 2011;11:8.

Perk J, De Backer G, Gohlke H et al.; ESC Committee for Practice Guidelines. European Guidelines on cardiovascular disease prevention in clinical practice (version 2012). *Eur Heart J* 2012;33:1635–701.

Scobie IN, Samaras K. *Fast Facts: Diabetes Mellitus*, 4th edn. Oxford: Health Press, 2012.

Smith SC Jr, Benjamin EJ, Bonow RO et al. AHA/ACCF secondary prevention and risk reduction therapy for patients with coronary and other atherosclerotic vascular disease: 2011 update: a guideline from the American Heart Association and American College of Cardiology Foundation endorsed by the World Heart Federation and the Preventive Cardiovascular Nurses Association. *J Am Coll Cardiol* 2011;58:2432–46.

Sniderman A, Durrington P. *Fast Facts: Hyperlipidemia*, 5th edn. Oxford: Health Press, 2010.

Steg PG, James SK, Atar D et al. Task Force on the management of ST-segment elevation acute myocardial infarction of the European Society of Cardiology (ESC), ESC Guidelines for the management of acute myocardial infarction in patients presenting with ST-segment elevation. *Eur Heart J* 2012;33:2569–619.

West R, Shiffman S. *Fast Facts: Smoking Cessation*, 2nd edn. Oxford: Health Press, 2007.

Combination antithrombotic therapy

Nearly one-third of patients with atrial fibrillation (AF) have coronary artery disease (CAD) and may need percutaneous coronary intervention (PCI) with stenting and long-term dual antiplatelet therapy (DAPT). As there is often a need for permanent anticoagulation in these patients, a combination of anticoagulation and DAPT (triple therapy) is recommended. In the vast majority, especially those with AF and an increased risk of thromboembolic events (e.g. $CHADS_2$ or CHA_2DS_2Vasc score of > 2; see *Fast Facts: Cardiac Arrhythmias*), triple therapy comprises acetylsalicylic acid (ASA; aspirin), a $P2Y_{12}$ receptor blocker (mainly clopidogrel) and a vitamin K antagonist.

Incidences of severe bleeding complications are greater with longer double or triple therapy administration: the risk of major bleeding in patients treated with triple therapy increases markedly at 1 year compared to DAPT (from approximately 2.4–2.8% to 12%). Therefore, antithrombotic combination therapy should be given only for the shortest possible time and frequently monitored to guarantee an international normalized ratio (INR) of 2–2.5. In this way, overall bleeding risk is reduced without an increase in major adverse cardiac events.

International guidelines. The European Society for Cardiology (ESC) has recently published its recommendations on antithrombotic combination therapy in patients with AF following coronary artery stenting (Table 7.1). These recommendations are based on individual bleeding risk (as determined by CRUSADE or HAS-BLED scores), the clinical entity at presentation (stable/elective patient or patient presenting with an acute coronary syndrome [ACS]), and the type of stent used (bare-metal or drug-eluting).

North American experts recommend a much longer duration of triple therapy than the current European approach in patients with

TABLE 7.1

European guidelines for antithrombotic strategies following coronary artery stenting in patients with atrial fibrillation

Hemorrhagic risk	Stent implanted	Recommendations
Low or intermediate	Bare-metal – elective	*1 month:* warfarin (INR 2.0–2.5) + ASA ≥ 100 mg/day + clopidogrel 75 mg/day + gastric protection *Lifelong:* warfarin (INR 2.0–3.0) alone
	Drug-eluting – elective	*3 (-olimus group) to 6 (paclitaxel) months:* warfarin (INR 2.0–2.5) + ASA ≥ 100 mg/day + clopidogrel 75 mg/day *Up to 12 months:* warfarin (INR 2.0–2.5) + clopidogrel 75 mg/day (or ASA ≤ 100 mg/day) *Lifelong:* warfarin (INR 2.0–3.0) alone
	Bare-metal/drug-eluting – ACS	*6 months:* warfarin (INR 2.0–2.5) + ASA ≥ 100 mg/day + clopidogrel 75 mg/day *Up to 12 months:* warfarin (INR 2.0–2.5) + clopidogrel 75 mg/ day (or ASA ≤ 100 mg/day) *Lifelong:* warfarin (INR 2.0–3.0) alone
High	Bare-metal – elective	*2–4 weeks:* warfarin (INR 2.0–2.5) + ASA ≥ 100 mg/day + clopidogrel 75 mg/day *Lifelong:* warfarin (INR 2.0–3.0) alone
	Bare-metal – ACS	*4 weeks:* warfarin (INR 2.0–2.5) + ASA ≥ 100 mg/day + clopidogrel 75 mg/day; drug-eluting stents should be avoided *Up to 12 months:* warfarin (INR 2.0–2.5) + clopidogrel 75 mg/ day (or ASA 100 mg/day) *Lifelong:* warfarin (INR 2.0–3.0) alone

ACS, acute coronary syndrome; ASA, acetylsalicylic acid (aspirin); INR, international normalized ratio.
Adapted from Lip GY et al. 2010.

low/moderate bleeding risk but increased stent thrombosis and stroke risk. For example, in cases where bare-metal stents are used, US guidelines recommend triple therapy for at least 6 months (similar to Europe), then an oral anticoagulant plus single antiplatelet therapy (ASA or clopidogrel) for 12 months, then oral anticoagulant monotherapy. In patients treated with drug-eluting stents, they recommend triple therapy for 12 months (6 months in Europe).

The biggest challenge for the near future will be the application of new anticoagulants and new more potent $P2Y_{12}$ receptor blockers in these currently recommended antithrombotic combination strategies.

Type of stent. In general, bare-metal stents or pure balloon dilatation are preferred over drug-eluting stents in triple therapy; drug-eluting stents should strictly be limited to special clinical and/or anatomic situations, such as long lesions, small vessels or diabetes where a significant benefit is expected. US guidelines recommend that drug-eluting stents should be totally avoided (and bare-metal stents used) in patients with an increased bleeding risk.

Other situations requiring triple therapy. Triple therapy is also used temporarily in patients with other reasons for permanent anticoagulation with vitamin K antagonists, such as patients with recurrent venous thrombosis/pulmonary embolism or artificial heart valves. However, there is no clear recommendation for these situations.

Gastric protection, preferably with proton pump inhibitors (PPIs), is recommended at least for the duration of the combination therapy. The use of PPIs, especially omeprazole, has been associated with a reduced pharmacodynamic effect of clopidogrel. This is because both clopidogrel and omeprazole are metabolized by the same hepatic CYP2C19 enzyme. Although the clinical significance of this interaction is not yet clear, guidelines recommend avoiding administration of clopidogrel and omeprazole except in certain conditions.

Site of access. In patients undergoing PCI under triple or dual antithrombotic therapy, radial access is preferred over femoral access to lower bleeding complications.

Personalized medicine in cardiovascular disease management

Since cardiovascular disease is influenced by multiple factors, optimal pharmacological management is dependent on both short- and long-term antithrombotic (antiplatelet and anticoagulant), antihypertensive and lipid-lowering therapies. However, most of these therapeutic regimens follow a 'one size fits all' strategy in common practice and as recommended by guidelines. These strategies do not account for individual differences in pharmacological response to these therapies and also genetic variations, particularly single nucleotide polymorphisms (SNPs) of genes associated with proteins responsible for the metabolism of these drugs.

Recent genome-wide association studies and pharmacological evaluation of cardiovascular drugs in individual patients have indicated an interindividual variation in drug response. In addition, translational research studies have linked this response variability to variable clinical outcomes, where patients with reduced drug response exhibit greater risk for adverse recurrent ischemic events. The latter findings have provided the foundation for personalized therapy in cardiovascular medicine, with the aim of providing patients with 'the optimal drug and dose at the right time'.

Antiplatelet therapy. Despite the fundamental importance of unblocked $P2Y_{12}$ receptors in the genesis of thrombosis, in general physicians do not objectively assess the intensity of the adenosine diphosphate (ADP)–$P2Y_{12}$ interaction in their high-risk patients treated with clopidogrel, and instead use a 'non-selective' or 'one size fits all' approach. This is paradoxical given the objective assessments and adjustments made after administration of most cardiovascular drugs; for example, weight-adjusted heparin is the standard of care in the USA for PCI, and the activated clotting time is used to determine an optimal level of anticoagulation.

Clopidogrel, the most widely used oral antiplatelet agent after ASA, is a prodrug that requires metabolic activation by P450 cytochromes (CYPs) to an active metabolite. Multiple lines of evidence suggest that variable and insufficient generation of active metabolite are the primary explanations for clopidogrel response variability and non-responsiveness, respectively.

Identification of high-risk phenotypes. The fundamental reason for genotyping clopidogrel-treated patients is to identify those with a high-risk phenotype, i.e. patients with high platelet reactivity. CYP isoenzyme activity is influenced by SNPs and also interactions with drugs (see below). Candidate gene studies conducted in healthy volunteers have demonstrated that loss-of-function polymorphisms of *CYP2C19* are associated with decreased exposure of the clopidogrel active metabolite and less platelet inhibition. The diminished effectiveness of clopidogrel in poor metabolizers (those with two loss-of-function *CYP2C19* alleles) has been recognized by the Food and Drug Administration (FDA) with a 'boxed warning' in the drug insert. Various meta-analyses of studies primarily involving PCI-treated patients have convincingly demonstrated an increased risk (approximately twofold) of the composite endpoint of cardiovascular death, MI or stroke among carriers of the loss-of-function allele when compared with non-carriers. However, trials of non-PCI-treated patients receiving clopidogrel have failed to demonstrate a significant association between *CYP2C19* loss-of-function allele carriage and adverse clinical outcomes. The relation of the gain-of-function allele (*CYP2C19*17*) carrier status, *ABCB1* genotype and paraoxonase-1 (PON-1) genotype to the antiplatelet response of clopidogrel and clinical outcomes in clopidogrel-treated patients are inconclusive at this time.

As noted above, clopidogrel metabolism is also influenced by concomitantly administered drugs (e.g. proton pump inhibitors, calcium-channel blockers, warfarin, cigarette smoke) that either interact or compete with clopidogrel during hepatic CYP450-mediated metabolism. Moreover, it has been reported that on-treatment platelet reactivity to ADP is influenced by the degree of CAD, age, gender, diabetes and obesity (Figure 7.1).

The net effect of all these influences is reflected in the final platelet reactivity phenotype. Thus, assessment of platelet function may be more appropriate than genotyping to indicate the risk of ischemic events, and genotyping alone may be considered in high-risk patients to determine the initial antiplatelet strategy.

Optimizing clopidogrel treatment. Numerous translational research studies conducted around the world, involving thousands of patients and multiple laboratory tests, have demonstrated that patients with high platelet reactivity are at increased risk for both short- and

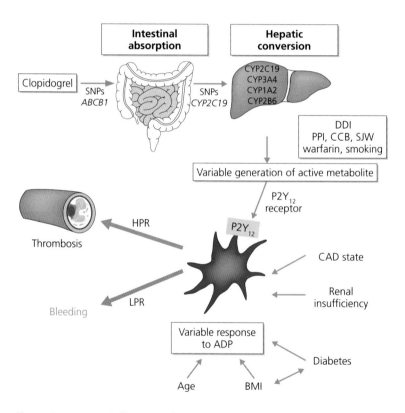

Figure 7.1 Factors influencing clopidogrel metabolism. BMI, body mass index; CAD, coronary artery disese; CCB, calcium channel blockers; CYP, cytochrome; DDI, drug-drug interaction; HPR, high platelet reactivity; LPR, low platelet reactivity; PPI, proton pump inhibitor; SJW, St John's wort; SNP, single nucleotide polymorphism.

long-term ischemic events after PCI, including stent thrombosis. Using different platelet function assays, cut-off values have been proposed for use in future studies of personalized antiplatelet therapy. Small early translational research studies have demonstrated that ischemic risk is not linearly related to on-treatment platelet reactivity but occurs above a moderate level of platelet reactivity to ADP. Similarly, recent observational studies have indicated that very low platelet reactivity is associated with bleeding. The concept of a 'therapeutic window' of $P2Y_{12}$ receptor reactivity associated with both ischemic event occurrence (upper threshold) and bleeding risk (lower threshold) has been proposed, similar to the INR range used for warfarin therapy, potentially allowing for personalization of antiplatelet therapy (Figure 7.2).

Prospective, albeit small, studies have provided evidence that high platelet reactivity is not just a diagnostic marker but a modifiable risk

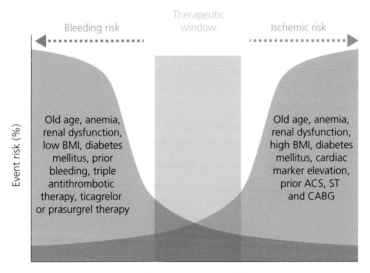

Figure 7.2 The concept of a therapeutic window for $P2Y_{12}$ receptor reactivity, below which bleeding risk increases and above which ischemic risk increases. ACS, acute coronary syndrome; BMI, body mass index; CABG, coronary artery bypass grafting; ST, stent thrombosis.

factor, where tailored antiplatelet therapy is associated with improved clinical outcomes in PCI-treated patients. However, conclusive evidence that personalized antiplatelet therapy improves clinical outcomes in patients with high platelet reactivity during clopidogrel therapy has not yet been demonstrated in a large-scale trial. In fact, it should be noted that the currently accepted cut-off values for high platelet reactivity have been associated in many studies with modestly increased odds ratios for ischemic events, high negative predictive values and low positive predictive values. However, given the overall low prevalence of thrombotic events in these studies, the low positive predictive values are understandable.

Moreover, there is debate about whether diagnostic test statistics have been appropriately applied to determine the utility of platelet function tests. The current data indicate that although platelet reactivity plays a major role in ischemic event occurrence, demographic and clinical factors must also be taken into consideration to optimally define the patients at greatest risk. A risk algorithm that includes biomarker testing with other clinical and demographic factors, similar to TIMI or GRACE risk scores (see Chapter 2), may improve risk prediction and guide physicians in the use of alternative therapies.

There are many gaps in our knowledge regarding the role of platelet function and genetic testing to optimize antiplatelet therapy, including:
- limited information on stable, non-PCI coronary disease patients
- few data on the relation of long-term platelet reactivity to both ischemic and bleeding events
- preliminary data only on the relation of phenotype and genotype to bleeding
- limited data on the utility of combining genotype and phenotype data for prognosis
- uncertainty regarding the variability of platelet function over time
- limited data relating platelet function to clinical outcomes in a major clinical trial of antiplatelet therapy.

Most importantly, there is limited evidence from large-scale trials that personalization of antiplatelet therapy enhances efficacy and improves safety.

Platelet function monitoring in patients undergoing surgery. The Society of Thoracic Surgeons recommend platelet function testing in high-risk patients undergoing PCI to determine the timing of surgery in patients receiving clopidogrel. The European and US cardiology guidelines recommend the withdrawal of clopidogrel therapy 5 days before surgery to allow platelet function to return to normal; therefore, testing may reduce unnecessary surgical delays in patients who have a suboptimal antiplatelet response to the drug.

Future perspectives. By assessing platelet function in all clopidogrel-treated high-risk patients, i.e. those with ACS (current or prior), a history of stent thrombosis and target-vessel revascularization, poor left ventricular function, multivessel stenting, complex anatomy (e.g. bifurcation, long or small stents), high body mass index and diabetes mellitus, and those co-treated with PPIs, patients found to be poor metabolizers of clopidogrel can be selectively treated with more potent $P2Y_{12}$ receptor therapy. Currently, unselective therapy with the new $P2Y_{12}$ receptor blockers is associated with increased bleeding. In addition, as clopidogrel is pharmacodynamically effective in about two-thirds of patients undergoing PCI, selectively treating two-thirds of patients with generic clopidogrel may provide significant cost savings. Recent European and US guidelines give a Class IIb recommendation to perform genotyping or phenotyping in high-risk patients undergoing PCI if the test findings will result in a change in antiplatelet therapy. In medically managed ACS patients, disease-related clinical risk factors seem to play a more pronounced role than on-treatment platelet reactivity.

Despite these debates, platelet function testing may have a role in monitoring the efficacy of clopidogrel as the chosen therapy and the safety of newer, more potent, drugs for long-term use, especially in low-risk patients and patients with a high bleeding risk. Platelet reactivity should not be regarded as an absolute and sole prognostic marker but should be evaluated in relation to patient risk, the timing of PCI and the presence of ACS. Future trials should evaluate the role of platelet function-guided approaches in preselected high-risk patients with clearly defined platelet-associated outcomes, and focus on the early phase after PCI. Preselection of high-risk patients and choice of potent active arms will be crucial to further define the role of personalized antiplatelet therapy. More differential approaches are warranted to use platelet function monitoring in combination with additional genetic and non-genetic risk factors to predict thrombotic and bleeding risks.

Antithrombotic therapy. Monitoring warfarin therapy based on INR to avoid risk of bleeding and thromboembolic complications is well established in clinical practice. Studies indicate that 20% variability in warfarin response is dependent on age, gender, bodyweight, diet, smoking status, concomitant medications and the presence of comorbidities, whereas 30–40% of variability in drug response is dependent on SNPs of genes encoding the CYP2C9 isoenzyme that is involved in warfarin metabolism and the *VKORC1* gene encoding vitamin K epoxide reductase. *CYP2C9*2* and *3* are the predominant SNPs of the *CYP2C9* gene, and their presence is associated with reduced CYP2C9 activity leading to slower warfarin metabolism. Therefore, carriers of the *2* and *3* alleles require a lower maintenance dose and cumulative induction doses. Similarly, numerous studies suggest that SNPs of the *VKORC1* gene have a significant influence on individual as well as ethnicity-dependent daily warfarin dose requirements, and personalized therapy based on genotyping may reduce the risk of bleeding. Despite lack of definitive evidence from a prospective study for improved clinical outcomes based on genotyping, the importance of genotyping in guiding warfarin therapy was acknowledged by the FDA in warfarin labeling in 2007.

Antihypertensive therapy. Demonstration of resistance to hypertensive drug therapies indicates that renin profiling may assist in personalizing antihypertensive strategies, and preliminary data suggest that such strategies may improve clinical outcomes. Similarly, haplotyping across renin-angiotensin-aldosterone and kininogen-kallikrein-bradykinin axes identify non-responders to angiotensin-converting enzyme (ACE) inhibitor therapies. However, there is a lack of strong evidence from randomized trials to implement these strategies in clinical practice.

Lipid-lowering therapy. Various statins at different doses have been shown to significantly reduce low-density lipoprotein (LDL) cholesterol, improving clinical outcomes, in numerous clinical trials. However, statin-induced myalgias in 3–10% of patients and continued cardiovascular events despite aggressive statin therapy indicate that personalized therapy may further improve clinical outcomes. Genetic polymorphisms of solute carrier organic anion transporter family member B1 (*SLCO1B1*) genes, which encode the organic anion-transporting polypeptide 1B1 (OATP1B1), may assist in identifying patients who are at risk of myopathy. It has been demonstrated that higher statin concentrations, particularly of simvastatin, are observed in subjects with a particular variant, *SLCO1B1*5*, indicating impaired influx transporter capacity.

Similarly, variants in the *APOA5* gene (encoding apolipoprotein A5) have been associated with hypertriglyceridemia, while the *NPC1L1* gene (the gene encoding the intestinal cholesterol transport protein Niemann-Pick C1 Like 1) has been associated with an exaggerated LDL-cholesterol response with ezetimibe. Personalization of lipid-lowering therapy based on these genetic analyses holds the potential to improve clinical outcomes.

Key references

Bhatt D, Scheiman J, Abraham N et al. ACCF/ACG/AHA 2008 expert consensus document on reducing the gastrointestinal risks of antiplatelet therapy and NSAID use: a report of the American College of Cardiology Foundation Task Force on Clinical Expert Consensus Documents. *J Am Coll Cardiol* 2008;52:1502–17.

Bonello L, Tantry US, Marcucci R et al.; Working Group on High On-Treatment Platelet Reactivity. Consensus and future directions on the definition of high on-treatment platelet reactivity to adenosine diphosphate. *J Am Coll Cardiol* 2010;56:919–33.

Degoma EM, Rivera G, Lilly SM et al. Personalized vascular medicine: individualizing drug therapy. *Vasc Med* 2011;16:391–404.

Gurbel PA, Mahla E, Tantry US. Peri-operative platelet function testing: the potential for reducing ischaemic and bleeding risks. *Thromb Haemost* 2011;106:248–52.

Huber K, Airaksinen KJ, Cuisset T et al. Antithrombotic therapy in patients with atrial fibrillation undergoing coronary stenting: similarities and dissimilarities between North America and Europe. *Thromb Haemostas* 2011;106: 569–71.

Lip G, Huber K, Andreotti F et al. European Society of Cardiology Working Group on Thrombosis. Management of antithrombotic therapy in atrial fibrillation patients presenting with acute coronary syndrome and/or undergoing percutaneous coronary intervention/ stenting. *Thromb Haemost* 2010; 103:13–28.

Mahla E, Suarez TA, Bliden KP et al. Platelet function measurement-based strategy to reduce bleeding and waiting time in clopidogrel-treated patients undergoing coronary artery bypass graft surgery: the timing based on platelet function strategy to reduce clopidogrel-associated bleeding related to CABG (TARGET-CABG) study. *Circ Cardiovasc Interv* 2012;5:261–9.

Subherwal S, Bach RG, Chen AY et al. Baseline risk of major bleeding in non-ST-segment-elevation myocardial infarction: the CRUSADE (Can Rapid risk stratification of Unstable angina patients Suppress ADverse outcomes with Early implementation of the ACC/AHA Guidelines) Bleeding Score. *Circulation* 2009;119: 1873–82.

Wijns W, Kolh P, Danchin N et al. Guidelines on myocardial revascularization: The Task Force on Myocardial Revascularization of the European Society of Cardiology (ESC) and the European Association for Cardio-Thoracic Surgery (EACTS). *Eur Heart J* 2010;31: 2501–55.

Useful resources

UK
British Atherosclerosis Society
www.britathsoc.org

British Cardiovascular
Interventional Society
Tel: +44 (0)20 7380 1918
bcis@bcs.com
www.bcis.org.uk

British Cardiovascular Society
Tel: +44 (0)20 7383 3887
enquiries@bcs.com
www.bcs.com

British Heart Foundation
Tel: +44 (0)20 7554 0000
www.bhf.org.uk

Cardiac Matters
www.cardiacmatters.co.uk

Heart UK
Helpline: 08454 505988
ask@heartuk.org.uk
http://heartuk.org.uk

UK Health Forum
Tel: +44 (0)20 7832 6920
www.ukhealthforum.org.uk

USA
American College of Cardiology
Tel: +1 202 375 6000
resource@acc.org
www.cardiosource.org

American Heart Association
Toll-free: 1 800 242 8721
www.heart.org
www.hearthub.org

Society for Cardiovascular
Angiography and Interventions
Tel: +1 202 741 9854
info@scai.org
www.scai.org

International
Asian Pacific Society of
Cardiology
Tel: +81 75 744 0007
secretariat@apscardio.org
www.apscardio.org

Asian Pacific Society of
Interventional Cardiology
Tel: +852 3109 7233
secretariat@apsic.net
www.apsic.net

Canadian Cardiovascular Society
Toll-free: 1 877 569 3407
Tel: +1 613 569 3407
info@ccs.ca
www.ccs.ca

Cardiac Society of Australia
and New Zealand
Tel: +61 2 9256 5452
info@csanz.edu.au
www.csanz.edu.au.com

European Atherosclerosis Society
Tel: +46 (0)31 724 2795
office@eas-society.org
www.eas-society.org

European Society of Cardiology
Tel: +33 4 92 94 76 00
www.escardio.org

GRACE 2.0 ACS Risk Calculator
App that provides the percentage
probability of death or death/MI at
time-points up to 3 years following
admission with an ACS
https://itunes.apple.com/gb/app/id6
87341279?mt=8&aff
Id=1736887

Heart Foundation (Australia)
Toll-free: 1300 36 27 87
www.heartfoundation.org.au

International Academy of
Cardiology
Tel: +1 310 657 8777
klimedco@ucla.edu
www.cardiologyonline.com

International Atherosclerosis
Society
www.athero.org

Medscape Cardiology/
TheHeart.org
www.medscape.com/resource/acs

Further reading – fastfacts.com
Other *Fast Facts* titles that may be
of interest include:
Fast Facts: Cardiac Arrhythmias
Fast Facts: Depression
Fast Facts: Diabetes Mellitus
Fast Facts: Heart Failure
Fast Facts: Hyperlipidemia
Fast Facts: Hypertension
Fast Facts: Obesity
Fast Facts: Smoking Cessation

Index

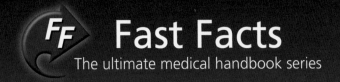

Our hope is that this Fast Facts *title helps you to improve your practice and, in turn, improves the health of your patients*

What will you do next?

Use this space to write some action points that have come from reading this book. And don't worry if you pass this on to a colleague, senior or junior; they are bound to find them interesting and may wish to add their own.

Action Point 1

Action Point 2

Action Point 3

If you have the time to share them with us, or you have suggestions of how to improve the next edition, we'd love to hear from you at feedback@fastfacts.com